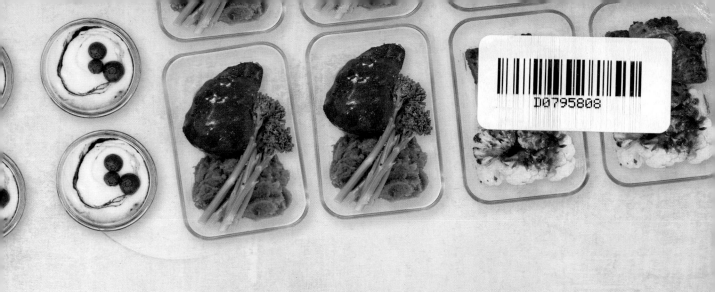

HEALTHY
MEAL PREP

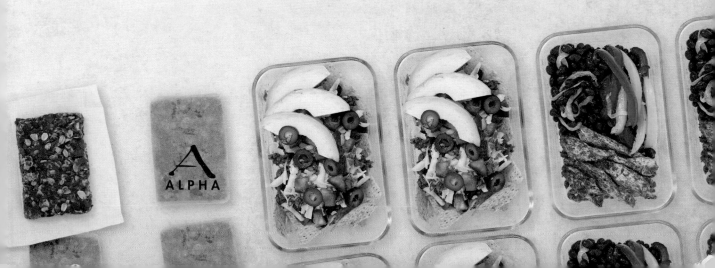

ALPHA

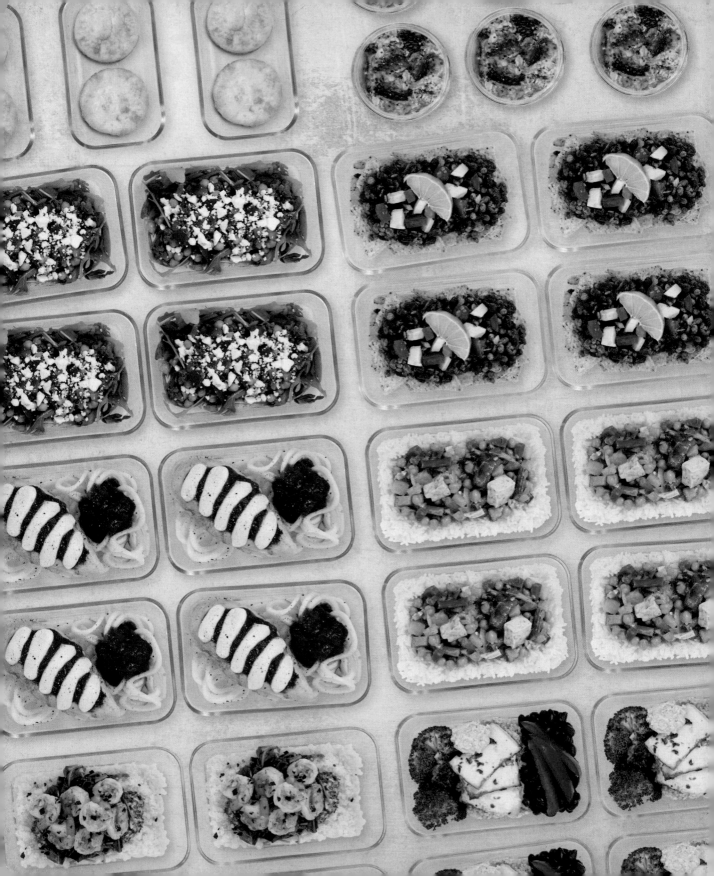

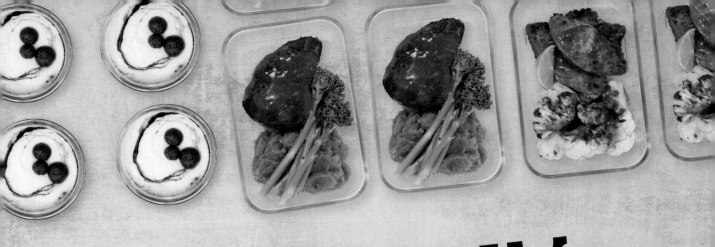

HEALTHY
MEAL PREP

time-saving **plans** to **prep** and **portion** your weekly meals

by **Stephanie Tornatore** and **Adam Bannon**
of **Fit Couple Cooks**

A
ALPHA

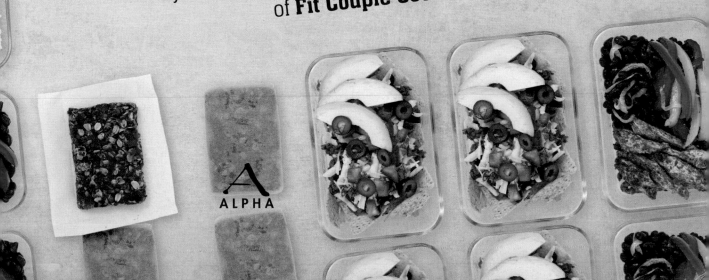

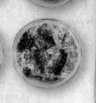
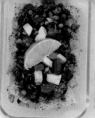
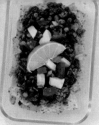
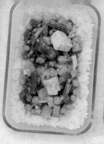
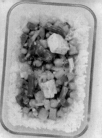
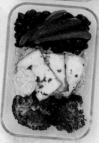
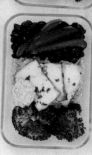

Contents

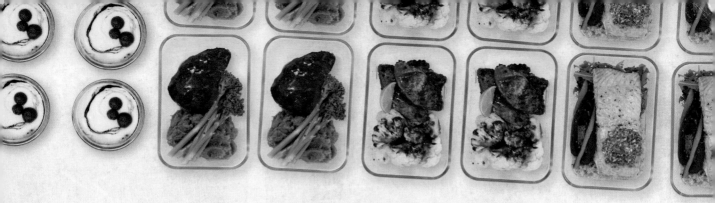

Introduction

With their YouTube channel, Fit Couple Cooks, Stephanie and Adam show fans how easy—and delicious—meal prep can be.

We started our YouTube channel Fit Couple Cooks because we're passionate about eating well, and we've seen first-hand the positive results of planning and preparing healthy meals in advance. After going through significant health transformations and losing a collective 100 pounds, we wanted to help others do the same. In less than two years, we've attracted over 400,000 people to join our Fit Couple Cooks YouTube family, and we've received thousands of comments from fans all over the world who have shed pounds and gained confidence just by switching to our meals. This book is an extension of that family, with complete meal plans and recipes to help you establish your own healthy meal prep habits.

With Adam's classically trained chef skills and Stephanie's creativity, we make simple, delicious recipes that are quick to prepare and provide a great balance of macronutrients. Meal prep doesn't mean giving up your favorite foods, and it doesn't mean eating chicken, broccoli, and rice three times a day. With our recipes, you can enjoy chicken nuggets, pad thai, and even lasagna!

In today's fast-paced world, we all make sacrifices to fit everything into tight schedules. But there is one thing you can never afford to sacrifice—your health. Meal prepping is the best way for busy people to eat good food and stick to health and wellness goals. To make it as simple as possible, we take care to develop our recipes using easy-to-find ingredients, basic kitchen equipment, and a minimum of pots and pans.

Our goals are to educate, inspire, and empower people to take control of their health—and it all starts with what's on your plate. Cooking for a whole week may seem overwhelming, but we promise, if you simply start meal prepping with these plans and recipes, you'll see just how easy it can be.

**Welcome to the Fit Couple Cooks family.
We are excited to have you join us!**

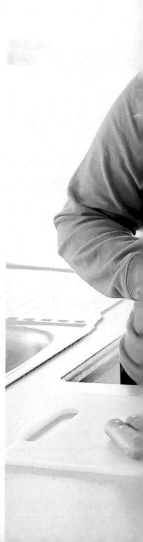

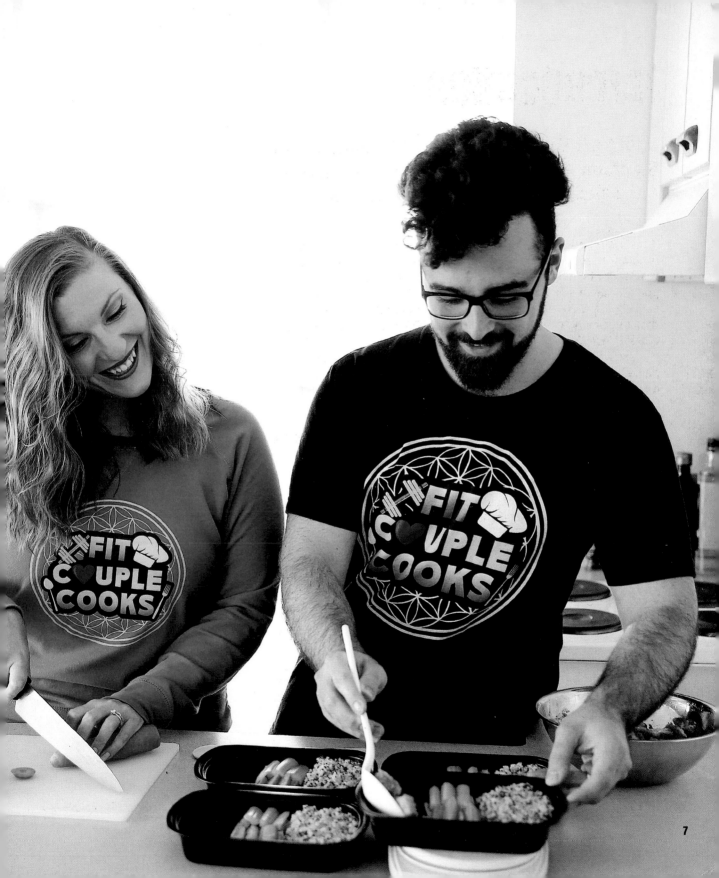

Why Meal Prep?

Preparing meals ahead is the best way to stay on top of your health goals and make the most of your time and money. You'll buy and eat food with intention instead of grabbing unhealthy meals on the go.

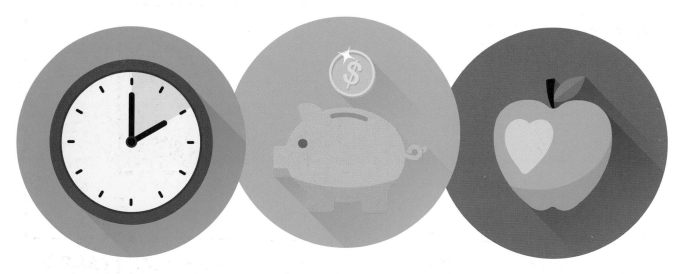

Save Time

Instead of preparing dinner from scratch each evening or scambling to make lunches in the morning, you can get your meals for the week ready in just a few hours on the weekend. Meal prepping for the week will take 2 to 3 hours, depending on the recipes. As with anything, the more you meal prep, the faster you will become.

Save Money

Meal prepping means no more expensive lunches out or last-minute takeout orders. With all of your meals prepared in advance, you'll have no reason to stop and buy something unhealthy on your way home. Customized shopping lists for each plan mean you won't overbuy food, and you won't throw away unused ingredients.

Eat Well

Having meals ready to go makes it more likely that you'll eat what you intend to eat, not what sounds good in the moment. This doesn't mean you'll only eat "diet food." It does mean that you'll have meals in reasonable portions, made with whole-food ingredients and balanced macronutrients.

How to Use This Book

1 **Choose a meal plan.**
There are 12 weeks of meal plans, and each week has recipes for four meals. These recipes make enough to feed one person for six days, leaving one day to eat out or cook something fresh.

2 **Check the shopping list and buy ingredients.** Each meal plan has a shopping list to make your trip to the store easier.

3 **Follow the Prep Day Action Plan.** A Prep Day Action Plan for each week guides you through preparing your meals.

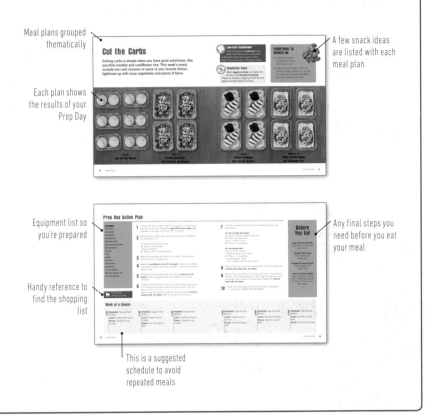

Meal plans grouped thematically

Each plan shows the results of your Prep Day

A few snack ideas are listed with each meal plan

Equipment list so you're prepared

Handy reference to find the shopping list

Any final steps you need before you eat your meal

This is a suggested schedule to avoid repeated meals

Won't I get bored eating the same thing every day for a week?

To keep things interesting, each plan in this book has one breakfast and three main meals, so you will be rotating your lunch and dinner every day.

What if I cook for more than one person?

You can either scale up the recipes as needed, or meal prep more frequently, every few days instead of once a week. You can also choose to use meal prep for only one or two meals per day.

What if I want to eat out?

You can! Meal prep will help you eat out when you want to, not because you have no other choice. Most recipes freeze well, so you can freeze a meal you didn't eat and enjoy it later.

What Makes a Healthy Meal?

Eating healthy doesn't mean having a salad for every meal. The recipes in this book focus on good-for-you ingredients and balanced macronutrients to help you achieve your goals.

Balanced Macronutrients

Macronutrients, or "macros" are the proteins, carbohydrates, and fats that make up the food we eat. All three macros play an important role in bodily function and are essential for good health. Every person has different macronutrient needs, depending on individual physique, activity level, and fitness goals. However, too often people shortchange themselves on protein and fat, and eat too many carbohydrates, especially those that hide in processed foods in the form of added sugar. The recipes in this book were developed with the goal of balancing the three macros, which is a healthy starting point for most adults. You can adjust the macro balance of your meals if needed.

Protein

Protein is made up of amino acids, which are essential for building and maintaining tissue. Good protein sources include meat, dairy, beans, nuts, and seeds.

Carbohydrates

The sugars, starches, and fiber in food are carbohydrates, and they are the body's primary energy source. Good sources include whole grains, vegetables, and legumes.

Fats

Although calorically dense, fats are the body's secondary fuel source and should not be avoided. Good sources include avocados, nuts, seeds, coconut oil, and olive oil.

Finding the Right Balance

Exact macro ratios vary by recipe, but aim to achieve a balance of protein, carbs, and fat.

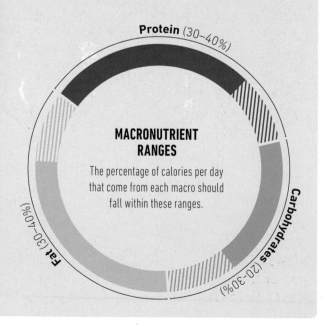

Protein (30–40%)
Carbohydrates (20–30%)
Fat (30–40%)

MACRONUTRIENT RANGES

The percentage of calories per day that come from each macro should fall within these ranges.

Reasonable Portions

It's easy to overeat, and just as easy to not eat enough. Pre-portioning your meals through meal prepping means you'll know exactly how much you're eating at each meal. Most meals in this book are between 400 and 600 calories and provide a healthy balance of macros, which prevents eating too many carbohydrates and not enough protein and fat. In addition to your prepared meals, be sure to eat snacks or a fourth meal each day to fully meet your calorie and macronutrient needs.

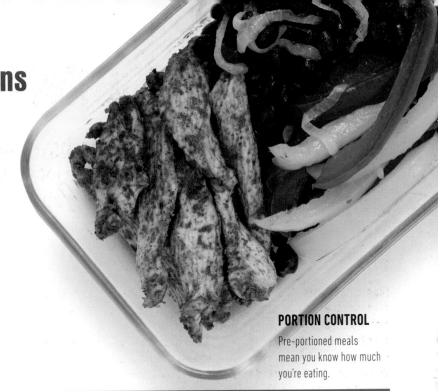

PORTION CONTROL
Pre-portioned meals mean you know how much you're eating.

Mindful Ingredients

The ingredients that go into your meals make a difference. These meals focus on lean protein and complex carbs, and avoid added sugar.

No refined carbs. Refined carbohydrates, like white flour, have been processed to remove the parts of the grain that are most nutritionally dense. The recipes in this book rely on whole-grain oats, rice, and corn, and avoid processed carbs, which makes most recipes naturally gluten free.

Low sugar. Most recipes have fewer than 10 grams of sugar per serving, and are sweetened with naturally occuring sugars in fruit and dairy rather than added sugars.

Healthy fats. You'll find lots of healthy fats, such as flaxseed oil, coconut oil, and olive oil, as well as raw nuts and avocados.

NATURALLY SWEET
Bananas and dates sweeten pancakes, muffins, and granola bars.

Meal Prep Must-Haves

Containers are essential for meal prep. For one person, you'll need 18 containers per week. It's helpful to have containers of the same size to simplify portioning and storing.

Plastic Containers

Pros: The most inexpensive option, plastic containers are light, stackable, and easy to store.

Cons: Plastic is less durable than glass or metal, and regularly heating plastic can cause it to break down. Plastic containers can't go in the oven.

What to look for: BPA-free containers that come in multi-packs for the best value.

Glass Containers

Pros: Durable and attractive, glass can be safely heated and will stand up to repeated use.

Cons: Glass is heavier and more expensive than plastic, and takes up more space.

What to look for: Shatter-resistant containers that can go from freezer to fridge to oven. Seek out lids with a rubber gasket and clips that lock on each side rather than one-piece plastic lids.

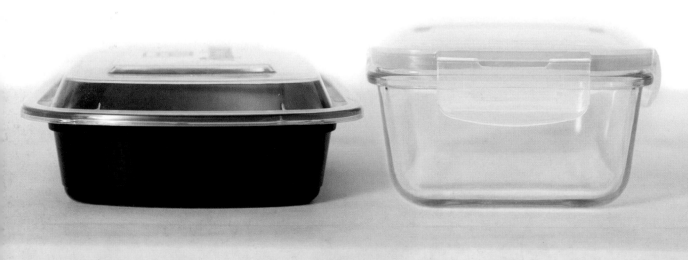

Other Equipment

The recipes in this book don't require much in the way of special equipment, but there are a few basic items that you'll need. The equipment list at the start of each Prep Day Action Plan lists the specific tools you'll need for the week.

- ○ Chef's knife
- ○ Cutting board
- ○ Mixing bowls
- ○ Measuring cups
- ○ Measuring spoons
- ○ Large sauté pan with lid
- ○ Saucepans
- ○ Pot with steamer insert

- ○ Baking sheets
- ○ Aluminum foil
- ○ Parchment paper
- ○ Mesh sieve or colander
- ○ Food processor or high-powered blender
- ○ Food scale (optional)

Metal Containers

Pros: Metal containers look great and are the most durable option.

Cons: The most expensive option. Metal containers cannot be used in microwaves and may not be suitable for use in ovens.

What to look for: Containers with latching metal lids rather than plastic lids.

Glass Jars

Pros: Small, lidded glass jars are inexpensive vessels for some breakfast recipes, like yogurt cups and overnight oats.

Cons: Jars may leak if lids aren't fitted tightly, and glass can break if dropped.

What to look for: Durable construction and tight-fitting lids. Glass canning jars with plastic screw-on lids are ideal.

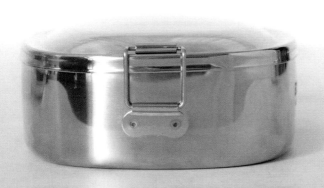

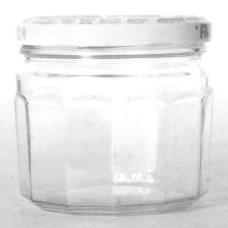

Storing and Reheating Meals

Once you've prepared a week's worth of meals, you need to know how to keep them tasting fresh and flavorful all week. All meals reheat easily and most can be frozen without compromising flavor or texture.

Fridge or Freezer?

Meals can be either refrigerated or frozen, depending on when you plan to eat them. Do not freeze fresh vegetables or toppings, such as leafy greens or raw tomato, as they will not thaw and reheat well.

Meat and poultry dishes: Refrigerate for up to four days, then freeze. Separate meat from any fresh ingredients before freezing. (Fresh toppings can be refrigerated separately for up to six days.)

Seafood dishes: Refrigerate for up to four days. Cooked fish does not thaw and reheat well, so freezing is not recommended.

Vegetarian dishes: Refrigerate for up to six days, then freeze. Remove any fresh toppings before freezing.

Keep meals refrigerated until ready to eat. Remove frozen meals from the freezer the day before you plan to eat them, and thaw in the refrigerator overnight before eating.

Get Ready to Serve

Many meals taste great when eaten cold, but if you want to reheat your meals, there are a few methods to choose from depending on your available resources.

Stovetop: Reheating on the stovetop is the best way to heat foods evenly and preserve texture. Most meals can be heated in a covered sauté pan for 3 to 5 minutes over medium heat. You may need to add a splash of oil or water to keep the food from becoming too dry.

Oven: To reheat a meal in the oven, transfer to an oven-safe dish and heat at 350°F (177°C) for 10 minutes, or until it reaches your desired temperature.

Microwave: You can microwave meals for 1 to 2 minutes, but it can result in uneven cooking and compromised texture. Microwaving plastic containers is not recommended.

Be aware that fish and egg dishes can easily become rubbery when reheated, so use a lower heat and take care not to heat for too long.

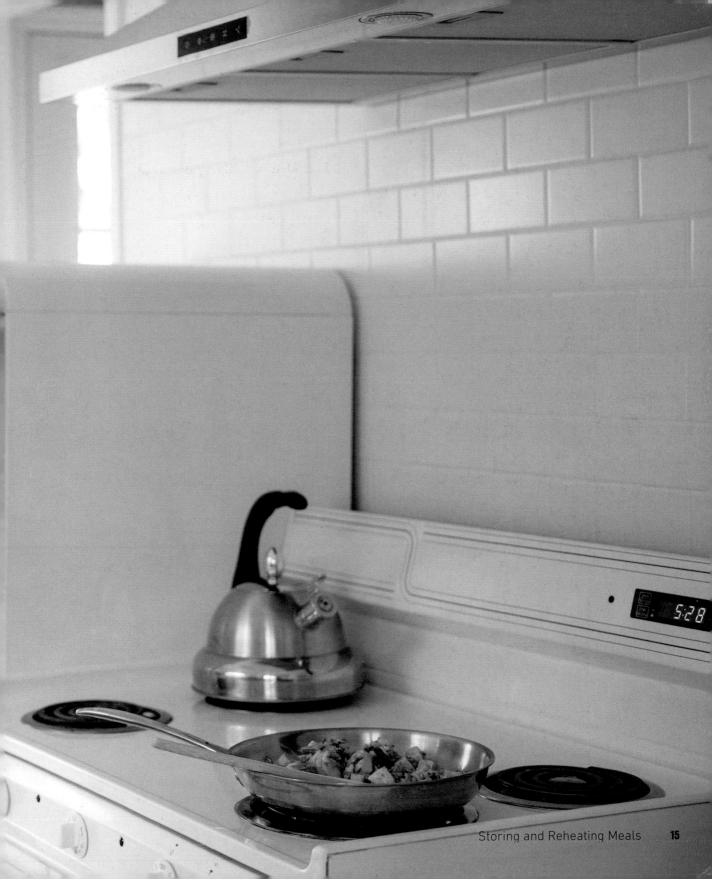

Fit Couple Cooks
Signature Sauces

Avoid added sugars and preservatives by making your own zesty and flavorful condiments.

BBQ Sauce

PREP TIME 5 minutes
COOK TIME 0 minutes

MAKES 1 cup
SERVING SIZE 2 tbsp

1 tsp garlic powder
½ tsp red pepper flakes
¼ tsp ground cloves
¼ tsp salt
¼ tsp freshly ground black pepper

1 tbsp olive oil
¼ cup apple cider vinegar
¼ cup tomato paste
2 tbsp Dijon mustard
3 tbsp water

1 In a medium bowl, stir together the garlic powder, red pepper flakes, cloves, salt, and pepper. Add the olive oil, apple cider vinegar, tomato paste, mustard, and water, and stir until well combined.

2 Transfer to an airtight container and refrigerate for up to 3 weeks.

NUTRITION PER SERVING
Protein 1g / Carbohydrates 2g / Fiber 0g / Sugars 2g / Fat 2g / Calories 30

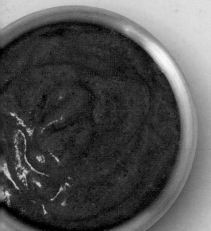

Quick Pesto

PREP TIME 5 minutes
COOK TIME 0 minutes

MAKES ½ cup
SERVING SIZE 2 tbsp

2 tbsp raw almonds
2 tbsp shredded Parmesan
Juice of 1 large lemon
2 garlic cloves, whole
2 cups fresh basil leaves, packed

¼ tsp salt
¼ tsp freshly ground black pepper
¼ cup olive oil

1 To the bowl of a food processor, add almonds, Parmesan, lemon juice, garlic, basil, salt, pepper, and olive oil. Process until smooth, pausing to scrape the sides as needed.

2 Transfer to an airtight container and refrigerate for up to 7 days.

NUTRITION PER SERVING
Protein 2g / Carbohydrates 2g / Fiber 1g / Sugars 1g / Fat 15g / Calories 151

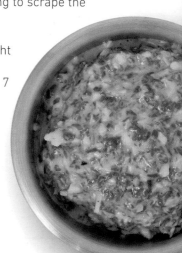

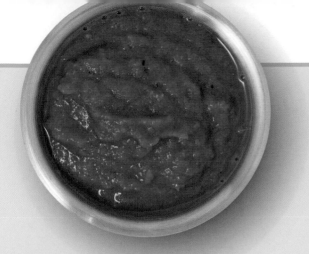

Ketchup

PREP TIME 5 minutes
COOK TIME 5 minutes

MAKES 3 cups
SERVING SIZE 2 tbsp

2 tbsp olive oil

½ medium yellow onion, diced

4 garlic cloves, minced

2 14.5oz (411g) cans diced tomatoes, drained

4 medium pitted dates, sliced, about 1oz (25g) in total

1 tsp salt

½ tsp freshly ground black pepper

1 In a medium saucepan, heat olive oil over medium-high heat. Add onion and garlic and sauté for 2 to 3 minutes.

2 Add tomatoes, dates, salt, and pepper. Increase heat to bring to a boil. Once bubbling, remove from heat.

3 Transfer the mixture to a blender or food processor and blend for 1 minute, or until mixture is smooth.

4 Transfer to an airtight container and refrigerate for up to 2 weeks.

NUTRITION PER SERVING Protein 1g / Carbohydrates 2g / Fiber 1g / Sugars 2g / Fat 1g / Calories 17

Buffalo Hot Sauce

PREP TIME 10 minutes
COOK TIME 30 minutes

MAKES 1 cup
SERVING SIZE 2 tbsp

¼ cup olive oil

1 medium yellow onion, diced

4 garlic cloves, minced

5 red chili peppers, such as cayenne, about 1½oz (40g) total, diced

1 cup water

1 tsp salt

1 tsp freshly ground black pepper

½ cup apple cider vinegar

1 In a medium pan, heat olive oil over medium-high heat. Add the onion, garlic, and chili peppers. Cook for 5 to 6 minutes until onions and peppers are soft and aromatic. Add the water and cook, stirring occasionally, for 10 minutes or until liquid has evaporated.

2 Transfer to a blender or food processor and blend for 10 seconds. Add the salt, pepper, and apple cider vinegar, and blend until smooth, about 30 seconds.

3 Pour the mixture through a mesh sieve to strain out the solids. Use a spatula to press out all of the liquid. Hot sauce can be refrigerated in an airtight container for up to 3 weeks.

NUTRITION PER SERVING Protein 1g / Carbohydrates 3g / Fiber 1g / Sugars 1g / Fat 7g / Calories 75

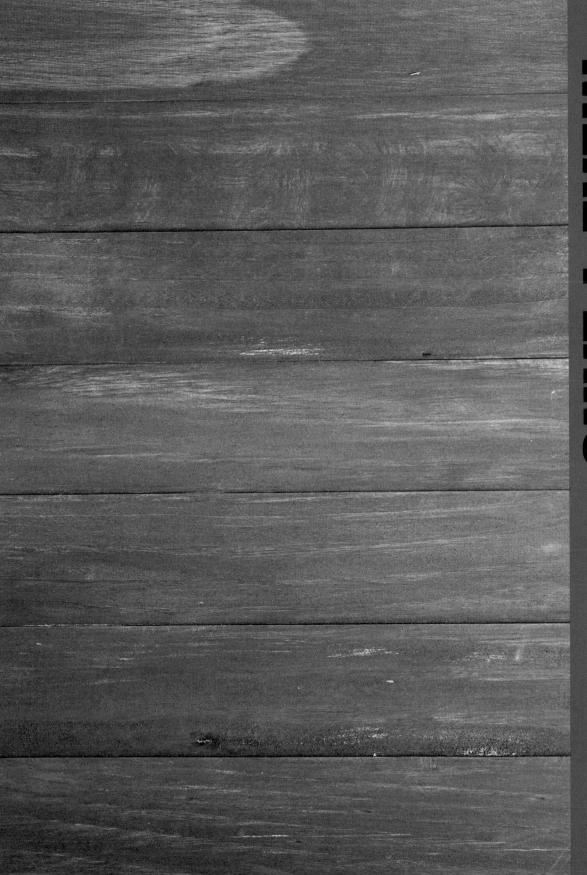

MEAL PLANS

Cut the Carbs

Cutting carbs is simple when you have great substitutes, like zucchini noodles and cauliflower rice. This week's meals include low-carb versions of some of your favorite dishes, lightened up with more vegetables and plenty of flavor.

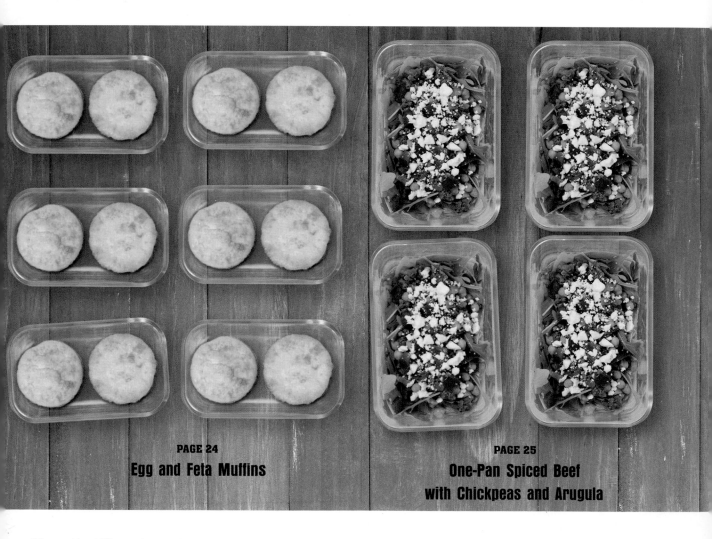

PAGE 24
Egg and Feta Muffins

PAGE 25
**One-Pan Spiced Beef
with Chickpeas and Arugula**

Low-Carb Cauliflower

Mild and adaptable, **cauliflower** is the perfect substitute for grain-based sides. A 100-gram serving has 5 grams of carbs, versus 23 grams of carbs in 100 grams of rice.

Vegetarian Swap

Meaty **eggplant slices** can replace the chicken in the **Chicken Parmesan.** Prepare as directed, swapping 3 thick slices of eggplant for each piece of chicken.

SOMETHING TO MUNCH ON

- Cheddar cheese slices are a filling low-carb snack.

- Keep raw almonds on hand to satisfy hunger pangs. A 1-ounce serving has 6 grams of protein and just 6 grams of carbs.

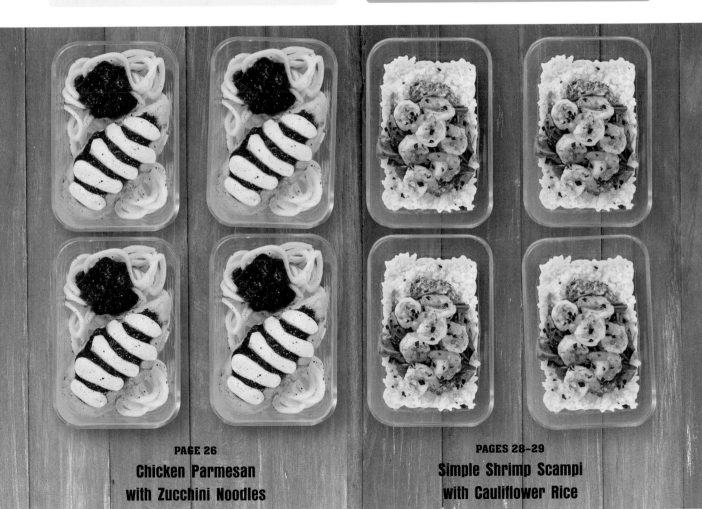

PAGE 26
Chicken Parmesan with Zucchini Noodles

PAGES 28-29
Simple Shrimp Scampi with Cauliflower Rice

Prep Day Action Plan

EQUIPMENT
Chef's knife

Cutting board

Mixing bowls

Measuring cups

Measuring spoons

Large non-stick sauté pan

Baking sheets (2)

Spiralizer

Tongs

Spatula

Mesh sieve

Food processor

Aluminum foil

12-hole muffin pan

Meal prep containers (18)

Food scale (optional)

 Cut the Carbs
shopping list, p142

1 Preheat the oven to 400°F (200°C) and grease a 12-hole muffin pan with coconut oil. Prepare the **egg muffins (p24, steps 1–4)** and place in the oven. Set a timer for 15 minutes.

2 While the egg muffins bake, wash and prepare the ingredients for cauliflower rice.

½ medium yellow onion, diced
➡ Place in a small bowl.
1 head cauliflower
➡ Place in bowl of food processor.

3 When the timer goes off, check on the muffins. Remove from oven and set on a cooling rack.

4 Make the **cauliflower rice (p29, all steps).** Divide the cauliflower rice evenly among 4 meal prep containers. Leave the lids off and allow to cool.

5 Rinse the food processor bowl and make the **pesto (p16, all steps).** Place 2 tbsp pesto over the cauliflower rice in each container.

6 Prepare ingredients for the shrimp. If using frozen shrimp, place in a mesh sieve and thaw under cold running water. Peel and devein shrimp if needed, and mince 4 garlic cloves. Wipe out the pan you used to cook the cauliflower rice, and make the **shrimp scampi (p28, all steps).** Add the shrimp to the containers.

Week at a Glance

Day 1
Breakfast Egg and Feta Muffins

Lunch Chicken Parmesan

Dinner Simple Shrimp Scampi

Day 2
Breakfast Egg and Feta Muffins

Lunch Simple Shrimp Scampi

Dinner One-Pan Spiced Beef

Day 3
Breakfast Egg and Feta Muffins

Lunch Chicken Parmesan

Dinner Simple Shrimp Scampi

7 Prepare ingredients for the chicken parmesan and one-pan spiced beef.

For the chicken parmesan:
4 medium zucchini squash, spiralized
➡ Place in a large bowl.
4 garlic cloves, minced
➡ Place in a small bowl.

For the spiced beef:
4 garlic cloves, minced
1 medium yellow onion, diced
➡ Place in a small bowl.
1 red bell pepper, diced
1 can chickpeas, drained and rinsed

8 Wipe out your pan, and line a baking sheet with foil. Prepare the **chicken parmesan (p26, all steps).**

9 Wipe out your pan. Measure 2 tsp ground cumin, 1 tsp mustard powder, 1 tsp smoked paprika, ½ tsp turmeric, ¼ tsp salt, and ¼ tsp pepper, and combine in a small bowl. Prepare the **spiced beef (p25, all steps).**

10 Divide the cooled egg muffins evenly among 6 containers (2 muffins per container) and refrigerate.

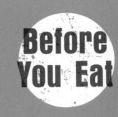

Before You Eat

Egg and Feta Muffins
Enjoy cold or briefly heat until warm.

Chicken Parmesan
Heat if desired, or enjoy cold.

Simple Shrimp Scampi
Heat if desired, or enjoy cold.

One-Pan Spiced Beef
Heat if desired, or enjoy cold. If reheating, separate the beef and beans from the arugula.

Day 4
Breakfast Egg and Feta Muffins
Lunch Simple Shrimp Scampi
Dinner One-Pan Spiced Beef

Day 5
Breakfast Egg and Feta Muffins
Lunch Chicken Parmesan
Dinner One-Pan Spiced Beef

Day 6
Breakfast Egg and Feta Muffins
Lunch One-Pan Spiced Beef
Dinner Chicken Parmesan

With just six ingredients, these grab-and-go breakfast muffins are a quick way to prepare eggs for the week.

Egg and Feta Muffins

PREP TIME 5 minutes **COOK TIME** 15 minutes **MAKES** 12 muffins **SERVING SIZE** 2 muffins

NUTRITION PER SERVING Protein 19g / Carbohydrates 3g / Fiber 0g / Sugars 1g / Fat 23g / Calories 295

3 tbsp olive oil

12 eggs

Salt and freshly ground black pepper

8oz (225g) full-fat feta cheese, crumbled

1 Preheat the oven to 400°F (200°C). Grease a 12-hole muffin pan with 1 tbsp olive oil.

2 Crack eggs into a large bowl, add remaining 2 tbsp olive oil, and season with salt and pepper. Whisk vigorously, until whites and yolks are well combined.

3 Place some crumbled feta cheese in each cup of the prepared muffin pan, and then pour the egg mixture over top, evenly dividing it among the 12 cups.

4 Place in the oven and bake for 12 to 15 minutes. The muffins are ready when they have doubled in size and are beginning to brown on top.
➡ *Return to Prep Day Action Plan while muffins bake.*

5 Remove from the oven and let cool in the pan. As the muffins cool, they will shrink and pull away from the sides. To assemble the meals, place 2 muffins in each of 6 meal prep containers.

TIP
Mix up these muffins by adding any vegetable or cheese of your choice.

Beef and chickpeas are cooked with peppers, onions, and spices and served over arugula for a filling meal.

One-Pan Spiced Beef
with Chickpeas and Arugula

PREP TIME 5 minutes   **COOK TIME** 15 minutes   **MAKES** 4 servings   **SERVING SIZE** 1 assembled meal

NUTRITION PER SERVING Protein 32g / Carbohydrates 14g / Fiber 4g / Sugars 4g / Fat 40g / Calories 544

¼ cup olive oil

4 garlic cloves, minced

1 medium yellow onion, diced

1 red bell pepper, diced

1lb (450g) ground beef or bison

2 tbsp tomato paste

2 tsp ground cumin

1 tsp mustard powder

1 tsp smoked paprika

½ tsp turmeric

¼ tsp salt

¼ tsp freshly ground black pepper

15oz (425g) can chickpeas, drained and rinsed

1 tbsp red wine vinegar

8oz (225g) full-fat feta cheese

4 cups baby arugula

1 In a large pan, heat olive oil over high heat. Add the garlic and onion. Sauté for 2 minutes, until onions are beginning to soften and garlic is fragrant. Stir in the bell pepper and continue to cook until onions are translucent.

2 Add the tomato paste and stir to coat. Add the ground beef, using a spatula to break up the meat. Cook until beef begins to brown, about 2 minutes, stirring occasionally.

3 Add the cumin, mustard powder, paprika, turmeric, salt, and pepper. Reduce heat to medium and cook for 3 minutes, stirring to coat the meat and vegetables with spices.

4 Add the chickpeas and stir. When the meat is fully cooked, add the red wine vinegar. Stir together and remove from heat.

5 To assemble the meals, divide arugula evenly among 4 containers. Top each bed of arugula with an equal portion of the beef and chickpea mixture. Top each meal with 2oz (56g) feta cheese, crumbled.

Replacing the traditional pasta with garlicky zucchini noodles lightens up this classic dish without losing the flavor.

Chicken Parmesan
with Zucchini Noodles

PREP TIME 10 minutes   **COOK TIME** 20 minutes   **MAKES** 4 servings   **SERVING SIZE** 1 assembled meal

NUTRITION PER SERVING Protein 48g / Carbohydrates 11g / Fiber 2g / Sugars 3g / Fat 37g / Calories 569

FOR ZUCCHINI NOODLES

¼ cup olive oil

4 garlic cloves, minced

4 medium zucchini squash, spiralized, about 1½lb (700g) total

FOR CHICKEN

2 tbsp olive oil

4 pieces skinless, boneless chicken breast, about 5oz (150g) each

Salt and freshly ground black pepper

8oz (225g) fresh mozzarella cheese, sliced

½ cup marinara sauce

1 To make the zucchini noodles, heat olive oil in a large non-stick sauté pan over high heat. Add garlic and sauté for 1 minute. Add the spiralized zucchini, cover, and cook for 2 minutes.

2 Remove the lid and toss the zucchini noodles with tongs, then cover and cook for another 3 to 4 minutes, until the zucchini begins to soften.

3 Transfer the zucchini noodles to a colander and drain. Spread the drained noodles on a baking sheet lined with paper towel, and press with additional paper towel to absorb excess moisture. Leave the noodles on the tray to dry.

4 To make the chicken, heat olive oil in a large non-stick sauté pan over high heat. Add the chicken, sprinkle with salt and pepper, and cook for 2 to 3 minutes. When the edges begin to turn white, flip them over and cook for another 2 to 3 minutes.

5 Transfer chicken to a foil-lined baking sheet. Spread 2 tbsp marinara sauce on each chicken breast and top with 2oz (55g) sliced mozzarella. Sprinkle with black pepper.

6 Turn the broiler to high and place the baking sheet in the oven, about 2 to 3 inches (5–7cm) below the heating element. Broil for 3 minutes, until the cheese is melted.

7 To assemble the meals, place 1 cup zucchini noodles in each of 4 containers and top with 2 tbsp marinara sauce. Add 1 piece of chicken to each container.

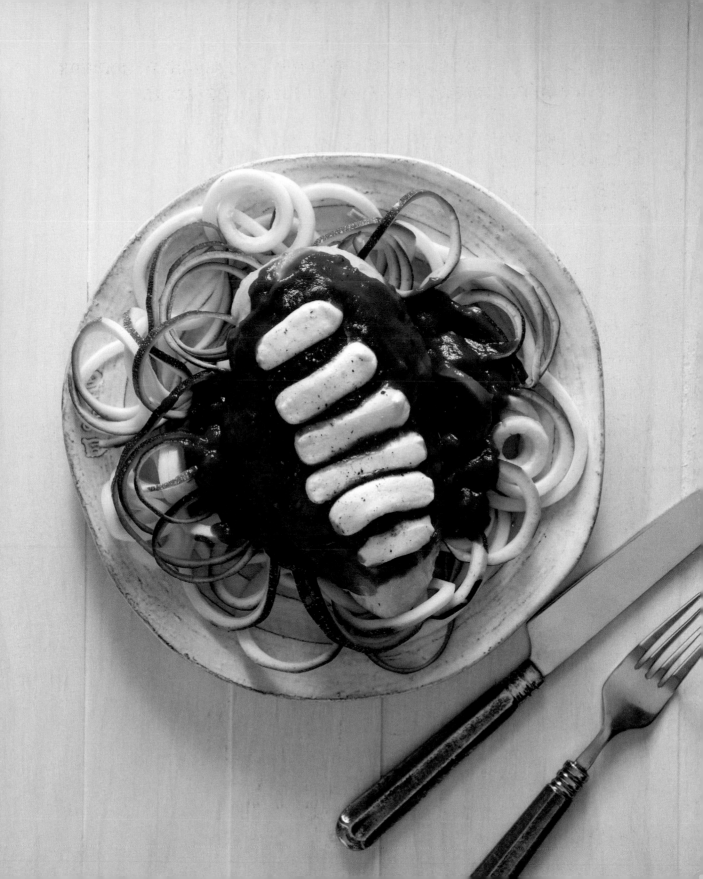

Shrimp is tossed in garlic, butter, and lemon and paired with cauliflower rice and zesty pesto in this twist on a classic.

Simple Shrimp Scampi

PREP TIME 5 minutes   **COOK TIME** 15 minutes   **MAKES** 4 servings   **SERVING SIZE** 1 assembled meal

NUTRITION PER SERVING Protein 42g / Carbohydrates 16g / Fiber 6g / Sugars 5g / Fat 40g / Calories 592

2 tbsp olive oil

4 cloves garlic, minced

1½lb (675g) raw medium shrimp, peeled and deveined

¼ tsp salt

¼ tsp freshly ground black pepper

1 tbsp dried parsley

1 tsp red pepper flakes (optional)

4 tbsp butter

Juice of 1 large lemon

4 cups baby spinach

4 cups **Cauliflower Rice** (see p29)

½ cup **Quick Pesto** (see p16)

1 In a large frying pan, heat olive oil over high heat. Add the garlic and cook, stirring occasionally, for 1 minute. Add the shrimp and cook until pink, about 2 minutes, turning with a spatula to coat the shrimp with garlic.

2 Reduce the heat to low and add salt, pepper, dried parsley, and red pepper flakes (if using). Stir to coat the shrimp with spices. Add butter and half of the lemon juice, and stir until butter has melted, forming a sauce.

3 Using tongs, transfer the cooked shrimp to a bowl, leaving the juices in the pan. To the same pan, add the spinach and cook, turning with a spatula until spinach has wilted, about 2 minutes. Add the remaining lemon juice and stir.

4 To assemble the meals, place 1 cup cauliflower rice into each of 4 containers. Top the cauliflower rice with 2 tbsp pesto. Divide the shrimp and spinach evenly among the containers and spoon any remaining juices over top.

This easy recipe transforms cauliflower into a satisfying low-carb substitute for cooked rice or pasta.

Cauliflower Rice

PREP TIME 10 minutes   **COOK TIME** 10 minutes   **MAKES** 4 cups   **SERVING SIZE** 1 cup

NUTRITION PER SERVING Protein 4g / Carbohydrates 12g / Fiber 6g / Sugars 6g / Fat 7g / Calories 127

1 head cauliflower, cored and cut into
   small florets, about 1¾lb (800g) in total

½ medium yellow onion, finely diced

2 tbsp olive oil

Salt and freshly ground black pepper

1 Place cauliflower in a food processor and pulse into rice-sized pieces. (You may need to work in batches, depending on the size of your food processor.)

2 In a large non-stick pan, heat olive oil over medium-high heat. Add the onion and sauté for 2 to 3 minutes.

3 Add the cauliflower and cook for 5 to 6 minutes, stirring occasionally. Season with salt and freshly ground pepper.

4 Remove from heat and allow to cool before transferring to an airtight container or using for meal prep.

Can I make a double batch to have extra on hand?

Yes, but it will need to be cooked in batches. If you make extra, you can store it in the refrigerator for up to 5 days, or freeze it.

Meal Prep Favorites

This week's meals feature some meal prep staples, including overnight oats and chicken, broccoli, and rice. These dishes are popular for a reason—they come together quickly, provide great nutrition, and are full of flavor.

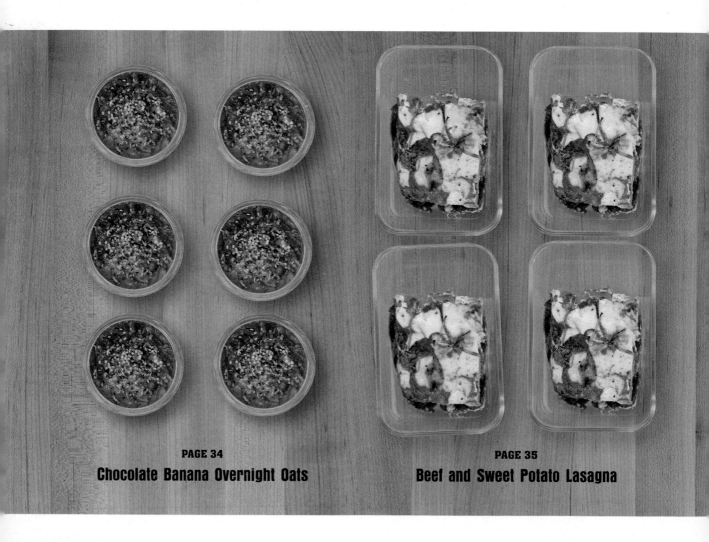

PAGE 34
Chocolate Banana Overnight Oats

PAGE 35
Beef and Sweet Potato Lasagna

Super Sweet Potatoes

Sliced or spiralized **sweet potatoes** can stand in for traditional pasta, and provide more nutrients instead of empty calories.

Vegan Swap

The **Chocolate Banana Overnight Oats** can easily be made vegan by using **almond milk** in place of cow's milk.

SOMETHING TO MUNCH ON

- Keep pre-cut red pepper strips in an airtight container in the fridge for easy snacking.

- Make some extra yogurt sauce (p36) to go with your red pepper strips or other cut veggies.

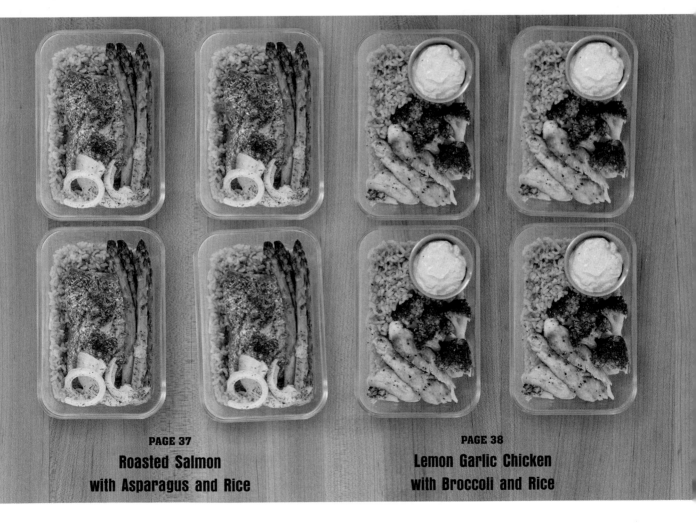

PAGE 37
Roasted Salmon with Asparagus and Rice

PAGE 38
Lemon Garlic Chicken with Broccoli and Rice

Prep Day Action Plan

EQUIPMENT

Chef's knife
Cutting board
Mixing bowls
Measuring cups
Measuring spoons
Large non-stick sauté pan
Medium saucepan
Baking sheets (2)
Aluminum foil
Mesh sieve
Spatula
Whisk
9 x 9in (23 x 23cm) baking dish
Small jars (6)
Meal prep containers (12)
Mandolin (optional)
Food scale (optional)

 Meal Prep Favorites shopping list, p143

1 Prepare rice for chicken and salmon meals. In a mesh sieve, rinse 1½ cups brown rice under cold running water until the water runs clear. Place rinsed rice in a medium saucepan, add 3 cups water, and stir. Cover and bring to a boil over medium-high heat. Once boiling, reduce heat to low and simmer for 15 minutes until the water has been absorbed.

2 While the rice is cooking, peel 2 sweet potatoes and slice into ¼-inch (.5cm) planks. (Use a mandolin for best results.)

3 Preheat the oven to 400°F (200°C) and begin preparing the **lasagna (p36, steps 1–3).** Once the beef sauce is simmering, check the rice. When the rice is cooked, remove it from the heat and let stand, covered, to cool.

4 Continue preparing the **lasagna (p36, step 4).** Put the lasagna on the bottom rack of the oven and set a timer for 30 minutes.

5 Once the lasagna is in the oven, line a baking sheet with foil and begin preparing vegetables for the salmon.

1 bunch asparagus, woody ends removed
1 medium yellow onion, sliced into half-moons
➡ Spread on the prepared baking sheet.

6 Prepare the asparagus and onion for the **salmon (p37, step 2).** Place the tray in the oven with the lasagna, on the top rack. Set a second timer for 10 minutes and clear your workspace.

Week at a Glance

 Day 1

Breakfast Chocolate Banana Overnight Oats

Lunch Lemon Garlic Chicken

Dinner Roasted Salmon

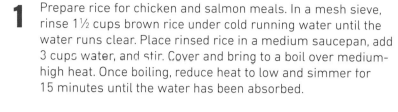 **Day 2**

Breakfast Chocolate Banana Overnight Oats

Lunch Roasted Salmon

Dinner Beef and Sweet Potato Lasagna

 Day 3

Breakfast Chocolate Banana Overnight Oats

Lunch Lemon Garlic Chicken

Dinner Roasted Salmon

7 When the second timer goes off, remove the vegetables and prepare the **salmon (p37, step 3).** Return the tray to the top rack. Reset the timer for another 10 minutes

8 While the salmon is roasting, prepare ingredients for the chicken and broccoli.

1lb (450g) chicken breast, sliced
4 garlic cloves, minced
➡ Place in a medium bowl.
1 head broccoli, cut into florets.

9 When the timer for the salmon goes off, remove the tray from the oven and set aside to cool.

10 Begin preparing the **chicken (p38, step 1).** When the timer goes off for the lasagna, remove the foil and return it to the oven. Set the timer for another 15 minutes.

11 While lasagna bakes, continue preparing the **chicken and broccoli (p38, steps 2–4).** When the timer goes off, remove the lasagna from the oven and set aside to cool.

12 Peel and dice 2 ripe bananas, and prepare the **overnight oats (p34, all steps).**

13 Portion the cooled lasagna and salmon into meal prep containers and refrigerate.

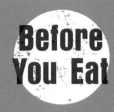

Before You Eat

Overnight Oats
Stir before eating and enjoy cold.

Lemon Garlic Chicken
Heat if desired. Top each meal with 2 tbsp yogurt sauce after heating.

Roasted Salmon
Heat if desired, or enjoy cold.

Beef and Sweet Potato Lasagna
Heat if desired, or enjoy cold.

Day 4
Breakfast Chocolate Banana Overnight Oats
Lunch Roasted Salmon
Dinner Beef and Sweet Potato Lasagna

Day 5
Breakfast Chocolate Banana Overnight Oats
Lunch Lemon Garlic Chicken
Dinner Beef and Sweet Potato Lasagna

Day 6
Breakfast Chocolate Banana Overnight Oats
Lunch Beef and Sweet Potato Lasagna
Dinner Lemon Garlic Chicken

This breakfast meal prep couldn't be easier. You're one bowl away from chocolate banana heaven, no cooking required.

Chocolate Banana Overnight Oats

PREP TIME 5 minutes | **COOK TIME** 0 minutes | **MAKES** 6 servings | **SERVING SIZE** 1 container

NUTRITION PER SERVING Protein 15g / Carbohydrates 30g / Fiber 4g / Sugars 8g / Fat 9g / Calories 261

2½ cups whole milk

1½ cups old fashioned (rolled) oats

2 tbsp hemp seeds

2 ripe bananas, diced

6 tbsp undenatured whey protein

2 tbsp raw cacao powder

1 In a large bowl, mix together the milk, oats, hemp seeds, bananas, whey protein, and cacao powder until well combined.

2 Divide the oat mixture evenly among 6 small jars or airtight containers. Refrigerate overnight before eating.

What is cacao powder? Can I use cocoa powder instead?

Don't swap cocoa for cacao! Cacao powder is the purest form of chocolate. It is raw and far less processed than cocoa powder.

Thinly sliced sweet potato takes the place of lasagna noodles in this Fit Couple Cooks fan favorite.

Beef and Sweet Potato Lasagna

PREP TIME 5 minutes   **COOK TIME** 1 hour   **MAKES** 4 servings   **SERVING SIZE** ¼ of pan

NUTRITION PER SERVING Protein 45g / Carbohydrates 25g / Fiber 5g / Sugars 7g / Fat 31g / Calories 559

1 tbsp coconut oil

2 garlic cloves, minced

1lb (450g) ground beef

2½ cups marinara sauce

2 tbsp dried Italian seasoning

2 medium sweet potatoes, peeled and sliced lengthwise into ¼-inch planks, about 10½oz (300g) in total

1½ cups whole milk ricotta cheese

2 cups baby spinach

1½ cups shredded mozzarella cheese

Salt and freshly ground black pepper

1 Preheat the oven to 400°F (200°C). In a large non-stick sauté pan, melt the coconut oil over medium-high heat. Add the garlic and cook for 1 minute, or until fragrant.

2 Add the ground beef to the pan, using a spatula to break up the meat. Cook until browned, stirring occasionally, about 5 minutes.

3 Add the marinara sauce and Italian seasoning and increase heat to high. When the sauce begins to bubble, reduce heat to low and simmer for 10 minutes.
➥ *Return to Prep Day Action Plan while sauce simmers.*

4 Line the bottom of a 9 x 9in (23 x 23cm) pan with slices of sweet potato. Top this layer with half of the beef mixture, then half of the ricotta cheese, half of the spinach, and half of the mozzarella, spreading each layer as evenly as possible. Repeat with the remaining sweet potato slices, beef mixture, ricotta, spinach, and mozzarella. Sprinkle salt and pepper over top and cover with aluminum foil. Bake for 30 minutes.
➥ *Return to Prep Day Action Plan while lasagna bakes.*

5 Remove the foil and bake, uncovered, for another 15 minutes, until the cheese is beginning to brown and the dish is bubbling at the edges. Refrigerate to cool completely before cutting.

6 To assemble the meals, cut lasagna into 4 equally sized servings and transfer to meal prep containers.

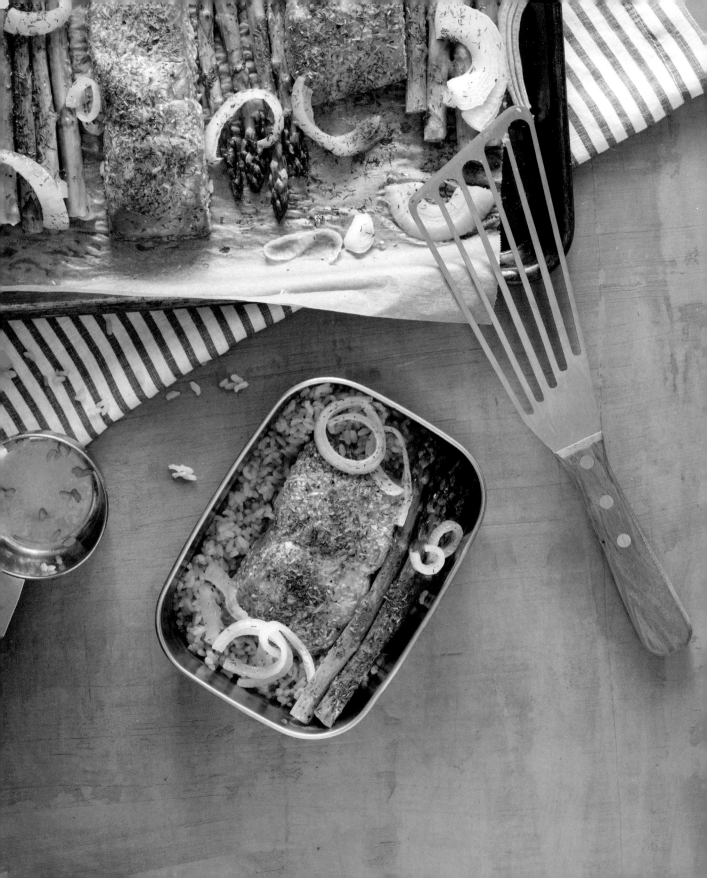

Roasting the onion, asparagus, and salmon on a single baking sheet makes this restaurant-worthy meal a snap to clean up.

Roasted Salmon
with Asparagus and Rice

PREP TIME 5 minutes   **COOK TIME** 20 minutes   **MAKES** 4 servings   **SERVING SIZE** 1 assembled meal

NUTRITION PER SERVING Protein 30g / Carbohydrates 30g / Fiber 5g / Sugars 4g / Fat 28g / Calories 492

1 bunch asparagus, woody ends removed, about 1¼lb (600g) total

1 medium yellow onion, sliced into half-moons

4 tbsp olive oil

4 pieces skinless salmon, each about 4½oz (125g)

Juice of 1 large lemon

1 tbsp dried dill

½ tsp salt

½ tsp freshly ground black pepper

2 cups cooked brown rice, to serve

1 Preheat the oven to 400°F (200°C). Line a baking sheet with parchment paper or foil.

2 Spread the onion and asparagus evenly across the prepared baking sheet. Drizzle with 2 tbsp olive oil and toss to coat. Place in the oven and roast for 10 minutes.

3 Remove the tray from the oven and arrange the salmon on top of the vegetables. Squeeze the lemon over the salmon and vegetables, and drizzle with the remaining 2 tbsp olive oil. Sprinkle the dill, salt, and pepper over top. Return the tray to the oven to roast for another 10 minutes, until salmon is lightly browned on top.
➡ *Return to Prep Day Action Plan while salmon roasts.*

4 To assemble the meals, place ½ cup cooked brown rice into each of 4 meal prep containers. Add an equal portion of asparagus and onions to each container, and top with 1 piece of salmon.

A spiced yogurt sauce and plenty of garlic and lemon make this classic meal-prep dish anything but bland.

Lemon Garlic Chicken
with Broccoli and Rice

PREP TIME 5 minutes   **COOK TIME** 30 minutes   **MAKES** 4 servings   **SERVING SIZE** 1 assembled meal

NUTRITION PER SERVING Protein 48g / Carbohydrates 32g / Fiber 5g / Sugars 3g / Fat 23g / Calories 527

FOR CHICKEN AND BROCCOLI

1½lb (675g) skinless, boneless chicken breast, sliced

4 garlic cloves, minced

Juice of 1 large lemon

¼ tsp salt

¼ tsp freshly ground black pepper

5 tbsp coconut oil

1 head broccoli, cut into florets

2 cups cooked brown rice, to serve

FOR YOGURT SAUCE

½ cup full-fat Greek yogurt

1 tsp ground cumin

¼ tsp cayenne pepper

1 Place the chicken in a bowl and add garlic, lemon juice, salt, and pepper. Stir to coat.
➡ *Return to Prep Day Action Plan while chicken marinates.*

2 In a large non-stick sauté pan, melt 1½ tbsp coconut oil over medium-high heat. Add half of the chicken to the pan and cook for 3 minutes, or until the edges begin to turn white. Flip the pieces and cook for another 3 minutes, until chicken is cooked through. Transfer cooked chicken to a shallow bowl. Melt another 1½ tbsp coconut oil and repeat with the remaining pieces of chicken.

3 In a medium pot, bring 4 cups water to a boil over high heat. Add the broccoli florets, reduce heat to medium, and cover. Cook for 6 minutes, until broccoli is bright green and crisp-tender. Drain the broccoli and return it to the pot. Add the remaining 2 tbsp coconut oil and toss to coat.

4 To make yogurt sauce, stir together the yogurt, cumin, and cayenne pepper in a small bowl. Transfer to an airtight container and refrigerate.

5 To assemble the meals, add ½ cup cooked brown rice to each of 4 meal prep containers. Add an equal amount of chicken and broccoli to each container, and pour any accumulated juices from the chicken over top. Serve with yogurt sauce.

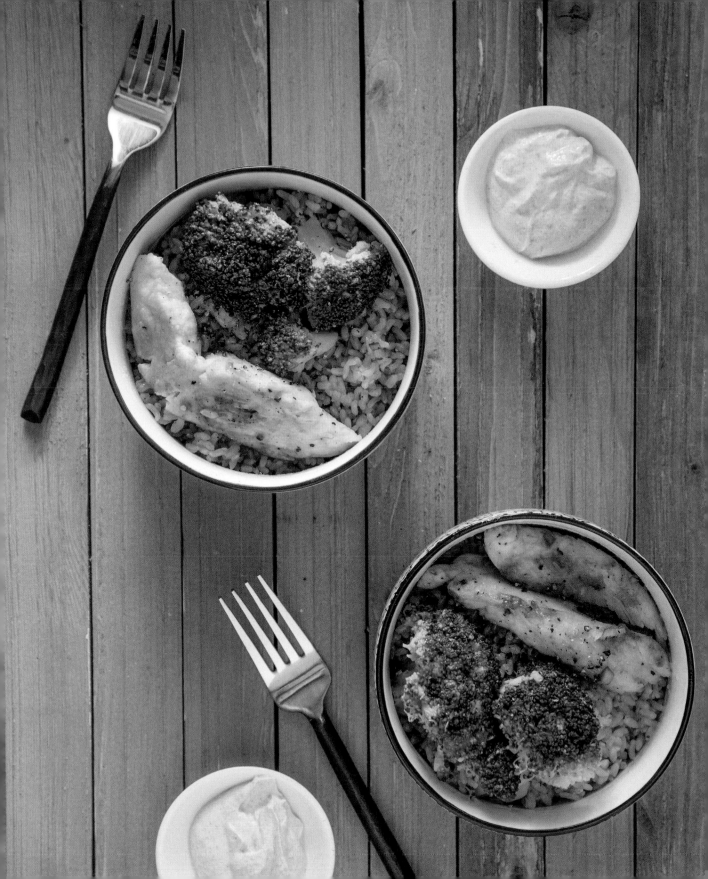

Healthy Game Day

Your favorite game-day foods don't have to be off limits. This week's meals include sports bar classics like beef nachos and Buffalo chicken, prepared without the processed ingredients and added sugar you usually find in these dishes.

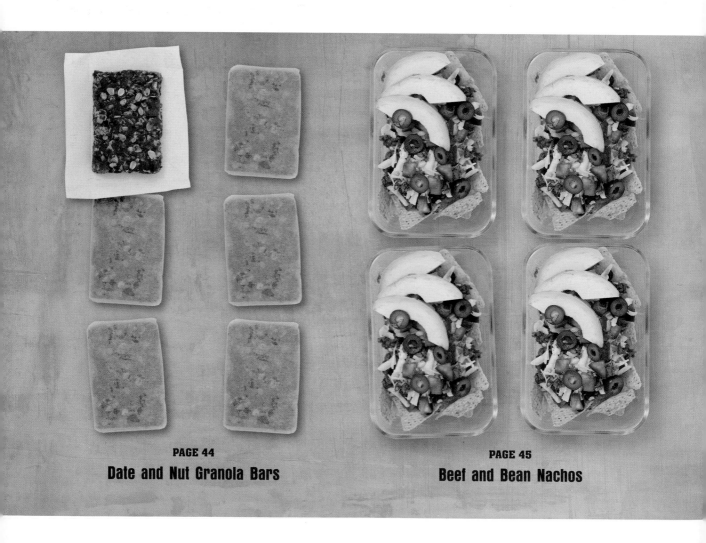

PAGE 44
Date and Nut Granola Bars

PAGE 45
Beef and Bean Nachos

Arrowroot Coating

Tossing cubed meat with **arrowroot flour** before cooking will help seal in flavor and moisture, and also add crispy texture.

Vegetarian Swap

Tender **cauliflower** can replace the chicken breast in the **Buffalo Chicken.** Prepare as directed, swapping 2lb (1kg) cauliflower florets for the cubed chicken.

SOMETHING TO MUNCH ON

- Supplement your meals with homemade popcorn. Sprinkle with olive oil, paprika, salt, and garlic powder for a Cajun twist.

- Cut some extra carrot and celery sticks and enjoy with almond butter throughout the week.

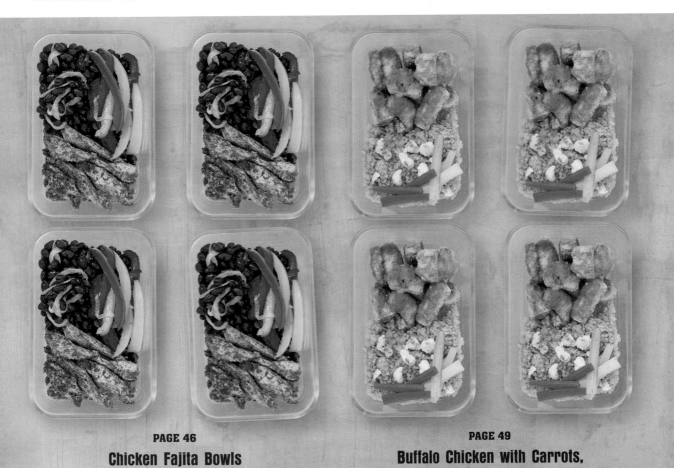

PAGE 46

Chicken Fajita Bowls

PAGE 49

Buffalo Chicken with Carrots, Celery, and Quinoa

Prep Day Action Plan

EQUIPMENT

Chef's knife

Cutting board

Mixing bowls

Measuring cups

Measuring spoons

Large non-stick sauté pan

Small saucepan

Medium saucepan

Baking sheets (2)

Silicone baking mats (2) or parchment paper

Aluminum foil

Mesh sieve

Spatula

Whisk

9 x 9in (23 x 23cm) cake pan

Food processor

Meal prep containers (12)

Food scale (optional)

 Healthy Game Day shopping list, p144

1 Prepare the **granola bars (p44, steps 1–8).** Then wash and prepare the produce for the remaining recipes.

For the hot sauce:
1 medium yellow onion, diced
4 garlic cloves, minced
2 red chili peppers, diced
➡ Place in a medium bowl.

For the buffalo chicken:
2 large carrots, cut into sticks
3 stalks celery, cut into sticks
➡ Divide among 4 meal prep containers.

For the fajitas:
1 large yellow onion, thinly sliced into half-moons
3 bell peppers, thinly sliced
➡ Spread on foil-lined baking sheet.

For the nachos:
1 large yellow onion, diced
2 tomatoes, diced
12 black olives, sliced
➡ Place each in a small bowl.

2 In a mesh sieve, rinse ¾ cup uncooked quinoa. Place in a medium saucepan and add 1½ cups water. Cover and bring to a boil over medium-high heat. Once boiling, reduce heat to low and simmer for 10 minutes until the water has been absorbed.

Week at a Glance

 Day 1

Breakfast Date and Nut Granola Bars

Lunch Beef and Bean Nachos

Dinner Chicken Fajita Bowl

 Day 2

Breakfast Date and Nut Granola Bars

Lunch Buffalo Chicken with Quinoa

Dinner Beef and Bean Nachos

 Day 3

Breakfast Date and Nut Granola Bars

Lunch Chicken Fajita Bowl

Dinner Buffalo Chicken with Quinoa

3 While quinoa cooks, cut up the raw chicken:
1lb (450g) skinless, boneless chicken breast, sliced into strips
1¼lb (600g) skinless, boneless chicken breast, cubed

4 Prepare the **hot sauce (p16, all steps).** While the peppers are cooking, check on the quinoa. Remove quinoa from heat when cooked and set aside. Reserve ¼ cup of the prepared hot sauce and refrigerate the rest.

5 Preheat oven to 400°F (200°C). While the oven heats, make the **buffalo chicken (p49, all steps).** Divide the cooked chicken and quinoa evenly among the 4 meal prep containers with the carrots and celery.

6 Begin roasting peppers and onion for the **fajita bowls (p46, step 2).** Set a timer for 30 minutes. Prepare the chicken for the **fajita bowls (p46, steps 3–4).** Place in the oven with the vegetables. The chicken will cook for 10 to 12 minutes.

7 While the vegetables and chicken are cooking, begin preparing the **nachos (p45, steps 1–2).** Once the beef mixture is finished simmering, the chicken should be ready to come out of the oven.

8 When the timer goes off, remove the peppers and onion from the oven. Finish by assembling the **nachos (p45, step 3)** and **fajita bowls (p46, step 5).**

9 Remove the chilled granola bars from the refrigerator, cut into 6 pieces, and wrap individually. Return to the refrigerator to store.

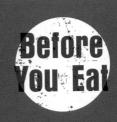

Before You Eat

Date and Nut Granola Bars
Keep refrigerated until ready to eat.

Buffalo Chicken
Remove carrot and celery sticks from container and heat chicken and quinoa, if desired.

Beef and Bean Nachos
Heat the beef and bean mixture, if desired. Add ½ avocado, sliced, and 1oz (28g) corn chips to serve.

Chicken Fajita Bowls
Heat if desired. Add ½ avocado, sliced, to serve.

Day 4
Breakfast Date and Nut Granola Bars
Lunch Beef and Bean Nachos
Dinner Chicken Fajita Bowl

Day 5
Breakfast Date and Nut Granola Bars
Lunch Buffalo Chicken and Quinoa
Dinner Beef and Bean Nachos

Day 6
Breakfast Date and Nut Granola Bars
Lunch Chicken Fajita Bowl
Dinner Buffalo Chicken with Quinoa

These lightly sweet, chewy bars are packed with whole-grain oats, nuts, and dried fruit to power your day.

Date and Nut Granola Bars

PREP TIME 10 minutes   **COOK TIME** 15 minutes   **MAKES** 6 bars   **SERVING SIZE** 1 bar

NUTRITION PER SERVING Protein 11g / Carbohydrates 39g / Fiber 5g / Sugars 20g / Fat 40g / Calories 560

20 medium pitted dates, about 5oz (150g) total

3 cups water

1 cup whole, raw, unsalted almonds, about 5oz (150g) total

1 cup whole, raw, unsalted walnuts, about 5oz (150g) total

1 cup old fashioned (rolled) oats

½ cup melted coconut oil

6 dried apricots, about 1½ oz (40g) total

1 Preheat the oven to 400°F (200°C). Line two baking sheets with silicone baking mats or parchment paper.

2 In a small saucepan, combine dates and water and bring to a boil. Once the water boils, remove from heat but do not drain.

3 In a food processor, pulse the almonds and walnuts until they are finely chopped, about 30 seconds.

4 Spread the ground nuts on a prepared baking sheet. Spread the oats on the second prepared baking sheet, and place both trays in the oven. Bake for 10 minutes, checking after 6 minutes to make sure nuts do not burn.

5 Drain the soaked dates and add to the food processor with coconut oil. Blend for 30 seconds, or until it forms a thick paste. Transfer dates to a large mixing bowl.

6 Add the apricots to the food processor and pulse until they are roughly chopped. Add to the mixing bowl with the dates.

7 Add the toasted nuts and oats to the dates and apricots, and mix to combine. Use your hands to bring the mixture into a ball.

8 Press the mixture firmly into a 9 x 9in (23 x 23cm) silicone pan or greased metal cake pan, using a spatula to create a smooth, even surface. Refrigerate for at least 2 hours.
➡ *Return to Prep Day Action Plan while bars chill.*

9 Cut into 6 bars and wrap each bar in wax paper. Refrigerate wrapped bars in an airtight container.

Balanced macros are the key to healthy nachos. This version has plenty of protein, so you won't overindulge on corn chips.

Beef and Bean Nachos

PREP TIME 20 minutes | **COOK TIME** 20 minutes | **MAKES** 4 servings | **SERVING SIZE** 1 assembled meal

NUTRITION PER SERVING Protein 36g / Carbohydrates 36g / Fiber 13g / Sugars 4g / Fat 40g / Calories 648

1 tbsp olive oil

1 large yellow onion, diced

1lb (450g) ground beef

1 tbsp tomato paste

1 tbsp chili powder

½ tsp garlic powder

1 tsp ground cumin

1 tsp smoked paprika

½ tsp salt

1 tsp freshly ground black pepper

8oz (220g) kidney beans (about ½ can), drained and rinsed

3oz (85g) shredded white cheddar

2 medium tomatoes, diced

12 pitted black olives, sliced

4 tbsp chopped fresh cilantro

2 avocados, sliced, to serve

4oz (112g) corn chips, to serve

1 In a large non-stick sauté pan, heat olive oil over medium-high heat. Add the onion and sauté for 2 minutes, or until fragrant. Add the beef, using a spatula to break up the meat. Cook until the meat has browned, about 3 to 4 minutes.

2 Reduce heat to low and add tomato paste, chili powder, garlic powder, cumin, paprika, salt, and pepper. Stir in the kidney beans. Simmer for 5 minutes and then remove from heat.

3 To assemble the meals, evenly divide the beef and bean mixture among 4 containers. Top each portion with an equal amount of shredded cheese, diced tomatoes, olives, and cilantro. Serve each meal with ½ avocado, sliced, and 1oz (28g) corn chips.

TIP
Package corn chips into individual plastic bags to keep chips crunchy and manage portion control.

These colorful bowls are brimming with Southwest flavor and packed with protein. You won't even miss the tortilla.

Chicken Fajita Bowls

PREP TIME 15 minutes   **COOK TIME** 30 minutes   **MAKES** 4 servings   **SERVING SIZE** 1 assembled meal

NUTRITION PER SERVING Protein 35g / Carbohydrates 29g / Fiber 12g / Sugars 5g / Fat 26g / Calories 484

1 large yellow onion, thinly sliced

3 red or yellow bell peppers, sliced into thin strips

2 tbsp extra virgin olive oil

Salt and freshly ground black pepper

1 tsp chili powder

1 tsp ground cumin

1 tsp smoked paprika

1lb (450g) skinless boneless chicken breast, sliced into thin strips

15oz (425g) can black beans, drained and rinsed

2 avocados, sliced, to serve

1 Preheat the oven to 400°F (200°C). Line 2 baking sheets with parchment paper or foil.

2 Spread the sliced onion and pepper on a prepared baking sheet. Drizzle with 1 tbsp olive oil and season with salt and pepper. Using your hands, mix the onions and peppers until they are evenly coated in oil. Place in the oven on the top rack and roast for 30 minutes.

3 In a medium bowl, whisk together the remaining 1 tbsp olive oil, chili powder, cumin, paprika, ¼ tsp salt, and ¼ tsp pepper. Add the chicken strips and toss to coat.

4 Arrange the chicken on a prepared baking sheet and place in the oven on the top rack (move peppers and onions to the bottom rack). Bake for 10 to 12 minutes, until chicken is fully cooked.
➡ *Return to Prep Day Action Plan while chicken and peppers cook.*

5 To assemble the meals, divide the black beans evenly among 4 containers. Add an equal amount of chicken and roasted vegetables to each container. Before serving, top each meal with ½ avocado, sliced.

TIP
To quickly deseed and slice peppers, cut off the top and bottom, then slice down one side. Remove the seeds, then cut into strips.

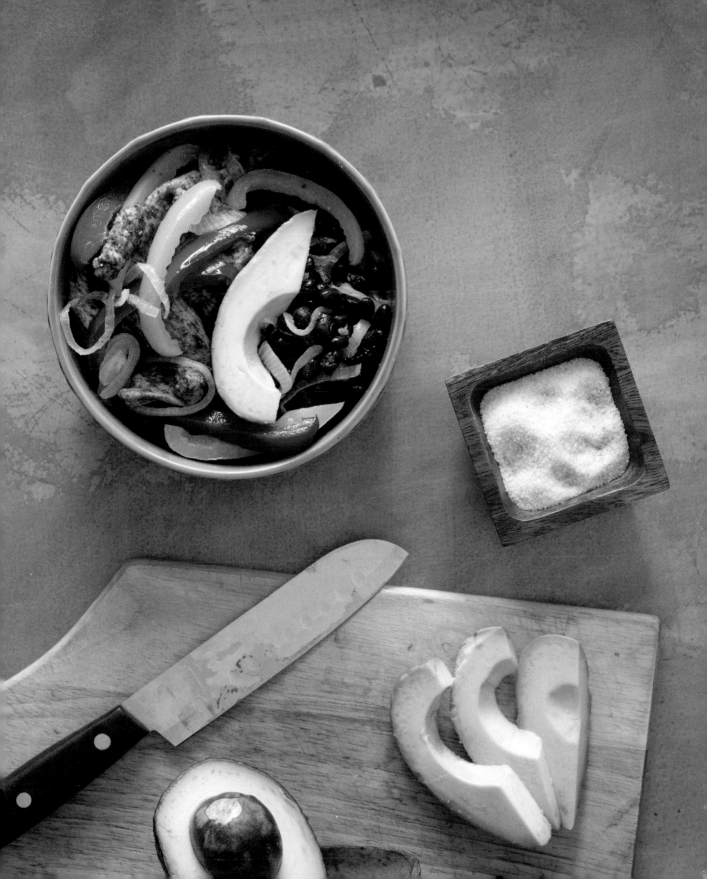

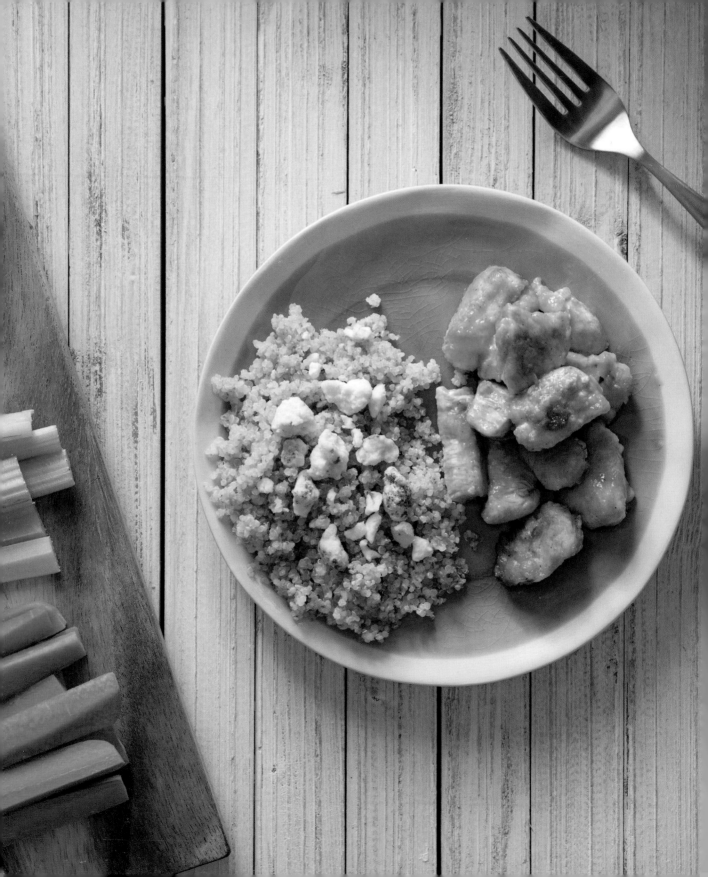

Tender chicken is coated in tangy hot sauce and served with quinoa for a healthy spin on this game-day favorite.

Buffalo Chicken
with Carrots, Celery, and Quinoa

PREP TIME 20 minutes   **COOK TIME** 20 minutes   **MAKES** 4 servings   **SERVING SIZE** 1 assembled meal

NUTRITION PER SERVING Protein 38g / Carbohydrates 38g / Fiber 4g / Sugars 2g / Fat 21g / Calories 493

1¼lb (600g) skinless, boneless chicken breast, cubed

½ cup arrowroot flour

¼ cup olive oil

¼ cup **Buffalo Hot Sauce** (see p17)

2 cups cooked quinoa

1 tbsp crumbled blue cheese

2 large carrots, cut into sticks

3 stalks celery, cut into sticks

1 In a medium bowl, toss together cubed chicken and arrowroot flour until chicken pieces are evenly coated.

2 In a wok or non-stick sauté pan, heat olive oil over high heat until shimmering. Add half of the cubed chicken and sauté for 2 minutes on one side, until golden brown. With a spatula, flip the chicken and sauté for another 2 minutes, until cooked through. Transfer the cooked chicken to a bowl. Repeat to cook the second batch of chicken.

3 Pour the hot sauce over the cooked chicken and toss until the chicken is evenly coated.

4 To assemble the meals, add ½ cup cooked quinoa to each of 4 containers and sprinkle with crumbled blue cheese. To each container, add an equal amount of chicken, along with carrot and celery sticks.

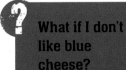

? **What if I don't like blue cheese?** You can omit the blue cheese or substitute any other soft cheese, such as goat cheese or feta.

Plant-Based Plates

You don't have to be vegan to enjoy meals without meat. This week's meals will show you how easy—and delicious!—it is to focus on plant-based foods, which are great for gut health. Bold flavors and plenty of filling protein will keep you satisfied.

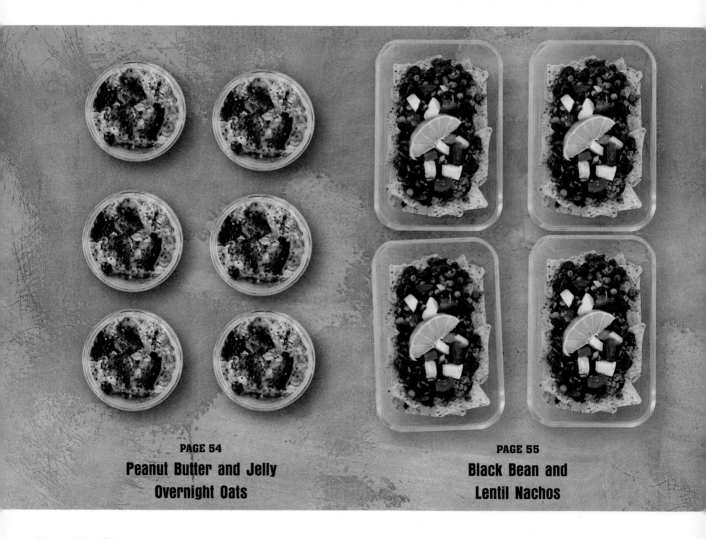

PAGE 54
Peanut Butter and Jelly
Overnight Oats

PAGE 55
Black Bean and
Lentil Nachos

Tasty Tofu

Versatile **tofu** is made from soybean curds. It is naturally gluten free, and is a great source of protein and calcium. Tofu will take on the flavor of any seasonings you use.

Omnivore Swap

If you can't go without meat for a week, just swap the **tofu** for an equal amount of **chicken** in the **Mixed Vegetable Curry.**

SOMETHING TO MUNCH ON

- Kale chips satisfy crunchy cravings. Drizzle kale with olive oil and roast at 425°F (218°C) for 10 minutes.

- Cut extra fresh veggies and make a double batch of hummus (p59).

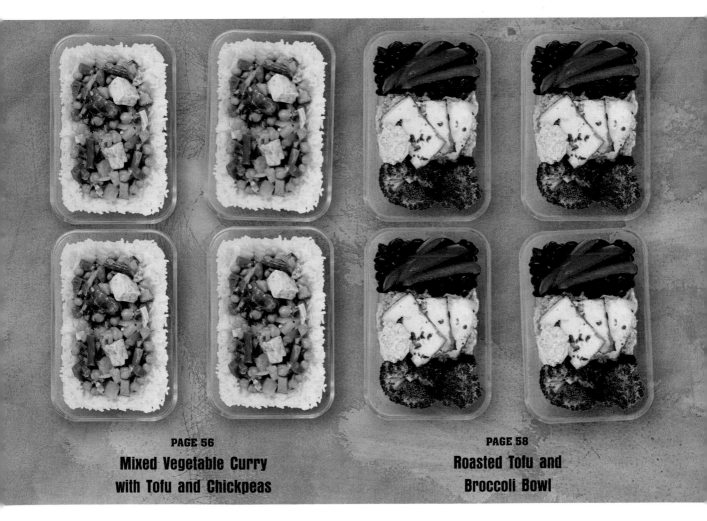

PAGE 56
Mixed Vegetable Curry with Tofu and Chickpeas

PAGE 58
Roasted Tofu and Broccoli Bowl

Prep Day Action Plan

EQUIPMENT

Chef's knife

Cutting board

Mixing bowls

Measuring cups

Measuring spoons

Saucepans (2 medium)

Wok or large, non-stick sauté pan

Baking sheets (2)

Mesh sieve

Silicone baking mats (2) or parchment paper

Food processor

Lemon juicer

Small jars (6)

Meal prep containers (12)

Food scale (optional)

 Plant-Based Plates shopping list, p145

1 Prepare rice according to package directions. You will need about ¾ cup uncooked basmati rice to yield 2 cups cooked.

2 While the rice cooks, dice 12 strawberries and prepare the **overnight oats (p54, all steps).** After the oats are prepared, check the rice. When the rice is cooked, set aside to cool.

3 Prepare quinoa according to package directions. You will need about ¾ cup uncooked quinoa to yield 2 cups cooked.

4 While the quinoa cooks, prepare the **hummus (p59, all steps)**. After the hummus is prepared, check the quinoa. When the quinoa is cooked, set aside to cool.

5 Preheat the oven to 375°F (190°C) and prepare ingredients for the tofu and broccoli bowls.

12oz (340g) tofu, sliced into 12 pieces
➡ Arrange on parchment-lined baking sheet.

1 head broccoli, cut into florets
➡ Place in a medium bowl.

4 garlic cloves, minced
➡ Place in a small bowl.

3 bell peppers, sliced
➡ Divide evenly among 4 meal prep containers.

Week at a Glance

Day 1

Breakfast Peanut Butter and Jelly Overnight Oats

Lunch Black Bean and Lentil Nachos

Dinner Roasted Tofu and Broccoli Bowl

Day 2

Breakfast Peanut Butter and Jelly Overnight Oats

Lunch Mixed Vegetable Curry

Dinner Black Bean and Lentil Nachos

Day 3

Breakfast Peanut Butter and Jelly Overnight Oats

Lunch Roasted Tofu and Broccoli Bowl

Dinner Mixed Vegetable Curry

6 Prepare the **tofu and broccoli (p58, steps 1–3).** Place in the oven and set a timer for 30 minutes.

7 While the tofu and broccoli roast, prepare ingredients for the curry. Drain and rinse 1 can of chickpeas, and cube 12oz (240g) tofu. Measure 1 tsp ground cumin, 1 tsp curry powder, 1 tsp turmeric, ½ tsp salt, and ¼ tsp pepper and combine in a small bowl. Wash and prepare produce.

1 small yellow onion, diced
4 garlic cloves, minced
1 piece ginger, peeled and minced
➡ Place in a small bowl.

1 medium carrot, diced
1 medium zucchini squash, diced
➡ Place in a medium bowl.

4oz (100g) green beans, cut into bite-sized pieces
3 mushrooms, sliced
➡ Place in a medium bowl.

8 When the timer goes off, assemble the **tofu and broccoli bowls (p58, step 4).** Then prepare the **curry (p56, all steps).**

9 Drain and rinse 1 can lentils and 1 can black beans. Dice 2 tomatoes and chop cilantro. Prepare and assemble the **nachos (p55, all steps).**

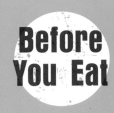

Before You Eat

Peanut Butter and Jelly Overnight Oats
Stir before eating and enjoy cold.

Black Bean and Lentil Nachos
Heat the bean mixture if desired. Add ½ avocado, sliced, and 1oz (28g) corn chips to serve.

Roasted Tofu and Broccoli Bowl
Heat if desired, or enjoy cold.

Mixed Vegetable Curry
Heat if desired, or enjoy cold.

Day 4
Breakfast Peanut Butter and Jelly Overnight Oats
Lunch Black Bean and Lentil Nachos
Dinner Roasted Tofu and Broccoli Bowl

Day 5
Breakfast Peanut Butter and Jelly Overnight Oats
Lunch Mixed Vegetable Curry
Dinner Black Bean and Lentil Nachos

Day 6
Breakfast Peanut Butter and Jelly Overnight Oats
Lunch Roasted Tofu and Broccoli Bowl
Dinner Mixed Vegetable Curry

Fresh strawberries and peanut butter bring all the sweetness you need to this simple and satisfying morning meal.

Peanut Butter and Jelly Overnight Oats

PREP TIME 10 minutes   **COOK TIME** 0 minutes   **MAKES** 6 servings   **SERVING SIZE** 1 jar

NUTRITION PER SERVING Protein 9g / Carbohydrates 22g / Fiber 7g / Sugars 2g / Fat 12g / Calories 232

2 cups unsweetened almond milk

1½ cups old fashioned (rolled) oats

3 tbsp chia seeds

12 strawberries, diced

6 tbsp all-natural peanut butter

1 In a medium bowl, mix together the almond milk, oats, chia seeds, strawberries, and peanut butter until well combined.

2 Divide the mixture evenly among 6 small jars or airtight containers. Refrigerate overnight before eating.

A flavorful seasoning mix turns humble canned beans into an addictive dip for corn chips, topped with tomato and avocado.

Black Bean and Lentil Nachos

PREP TIME 10 minutes   **COOK TIME** 0 minutes   **MAKES** 4 servings   **SERVING SIZE** 1 assembled meal

NUTRITION PER SERVING Protein 17g / Carbohydrates 56g / Fiber 16g / Sugars 2g / Fat 31g / Calories 571

2 tbsp olive oil

1 tbsp red wine vinegar

2 tbsp tomato paste

1 tbsp chili powder

½ tsp salt

½ tsp freshly ground black pepper

15oz (425g) can lentils, drained and rinsed

15oz (425g) can black beans, drained and rinsed

¼ cup chopped fresh cilantro (optional)

2 medium tomatoes, diced

1 lime, quartered

2 avocados, cubed, to serve

4oz (112g) corn chips, to serve

1 In a large bowl, whisk together olive oil, red wine vinegar, tomato paste, chili powder, salt, and pepper. Add the lentils, black beans, and cilantro, if using. Stir together until well combined.

2 To assemble the meals, divide the bean mixture evenly among 4 containers. Add an equal amount of diced tomato and cilantro, if using, to each meal, and top with a lime wedge. Serve each meal with ½ avocado, cubed, and 1oz (28g) corn chips.

TIP
Add shredded cheese —vegan or regular— to your nachos if desired.

This one-pan meal is flavored with an aromatic blend of cumin, curry, and turmeric and served over fluffy rice.

Mixed Vegetable Curry
with Tofu and Chickpeas

PREP TIME 15 minutes　　**COOK TIME** 15 minutes　　**MAKES** 4 servings　　**SERVING SIZE** 1 assembled meal

NUTRITION PER SERVING Protein 22g / Carbohydrates 46g / Fiber 9g / Sugars 5g / Fat 34g / Calories 578

2 tbsp coconut oil

1 small yellow onion, diced

4 garlic cloves, minced

Small piece of ginger, peeled and minced

1 medium carrot, diced

1 medium zucchini squash, diced

4oz (100g) green beans, trimmed and cut into bite-size pieces

3 large mushrooms, sliced, about 4oz (100g) in total

15oz (425g) can chickpeas

12oz (340g) extra firm tofu, cubed

13.5oz (398g) can full-fat coconut milk

1 tsp ground cumin

1 tsp curry powder

1 tsp turmeric

½ tsp salt

¼ tsp freshly ground black pepper

2 cups cooked basmati rice

1 In large, non-stick sauté pan, melt coconut oil over high heat. Add the onion, garlic, and ginger, and sauté for 2 minutes or until fragrant, stirring frequently. Reduce heat to medium-high.

2 Add the carrot and zucchini and cook for 2 minutes. Add the green beans and mushrooms and cook for another 2 minutes. When the mushrooms begin to brown, add the chickpeas and tofu and cook for 2 minutes more.

3 Add the coconut milk, cumin, curry powder, turmeric, salt, and pepper. Stir together and bring to a boil. Once boiling, remove from heat and cool for a few minutes.

4 To assemble the meals, add ½ cup cooked basmati rice to each of 4 meal prep containers. Scoop the curry over the rice, dividing it evenly among the containers.

TIP
Almost any vegetable can be added to this adaptable curry.

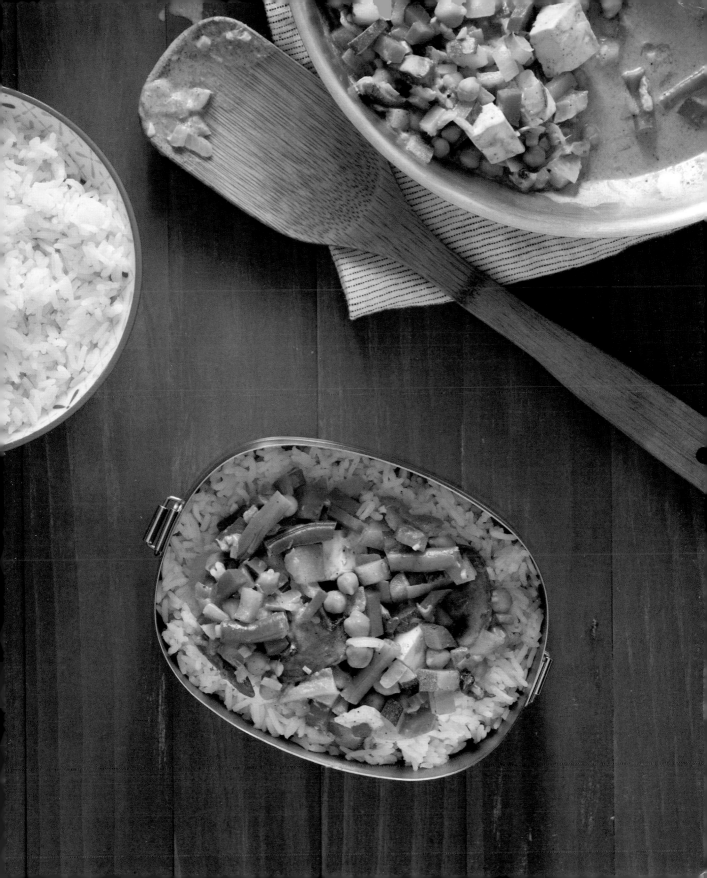

Tofu is roasted with garlic and lemon and accompanied by broccoli, quinoa, black beans, and peppers in this robust bowl.

Roasted Tofu and Broccoli Bowl

PREP TIME 10 minutes   **COOK TIME** 30 minutes   **MAKES** 4 servings   **SERVING SIZE** 1 assembled meal

NUTRITION PER SERVING Protein 30g / Carbohydrates 55g / Fiber 12g / Sugars 6g / Fat 30g / Calories 610

4 garlic cloves, minced

Juice of 1 lemon

4 tbsp olive oil

1 head broccoli, cut into florets

12oz (340g) extra firm tofu, cut into 12 slices

2 cups cooked quinoa

3 red bell peppers, cut into strips

15oz (425g) can black beans, drained and rinsed

½ cup **Hummus** (see p59)

Chopped cilantro, for garnish (optional)

1 Preheat the oven to 375°F (190°C) and line 2 baking sheets with silicone baking mats or parchment paper.

2 In a small bowl, whisk together the garlic, juice of ½ lemon, and 2 tbsp olive oil. Arrange the tofu slices on a prepared baking sheet and brush the tofu with the lemon garlic mixture.

3 In a medium bowl, toss broccoli florets with the juice of the remaining ½ lemon and remaining 2 tbsp olive oil until well-coated. Spread on the second prepared baking sheet. Place the tray of broccoli and the tray of tofu in the oven. Bake both trays for 30 minutes.
➡ *Return to Prep Day Action Plan while tofu and broccoli roast.*

4 To assemble the meals, place ½ cup cooked quinoa in each of 4 meal prep containers. Add 3 pieces of tofu to each container, along with an equal portion of cooked broccoli, sliced bell pepper, and black beans. Finish by adding 2 tbsp hummus to each container, and garnish with chopped cilantro, if using.

This simple recipe comes together quickly. Have some ready to go in your fridge for whenever hunger strikes.

Hummus

PREP TIME 5 minutes **COOK TIME** 0 minutes **MAKES** 1 cup **SERVING SIZE** 2 tbsp

NUTRITION PER SERVING Protein 5g / Carbohydrates 10g / Fiber 3g / Sugars 0g / Fat 9g / Calories 141

2 tbsp olive oil

Juice of ½ lemon

2 garlic cloves, peeled

1 tbsp sesame seeds

15oz (425g) can chickpeas, drained and rinsed

¼ tsp salt

¼ tsp freshly ground black pepper

1 In the bowl of a food processor or high-powered blender, combine all ingredients and process until smooth, adding up to 3 tbsp water as needed to achieve the desired consistency. Taste and season with salt and pepper if needed.

2 Transfer hummus to an airtight container and refrigerate for up to 7 days. The hummus tastes best a day or two after it's made.

Cozy Comfort Food

If the weather is chilly or you have a stressful week ahead, you need comfort food—but it doesn't have to be unhealthy. Grown-up versions of childhood favorites like chicken nuggets, pancakes, and chili will have you feeling cozy all week.

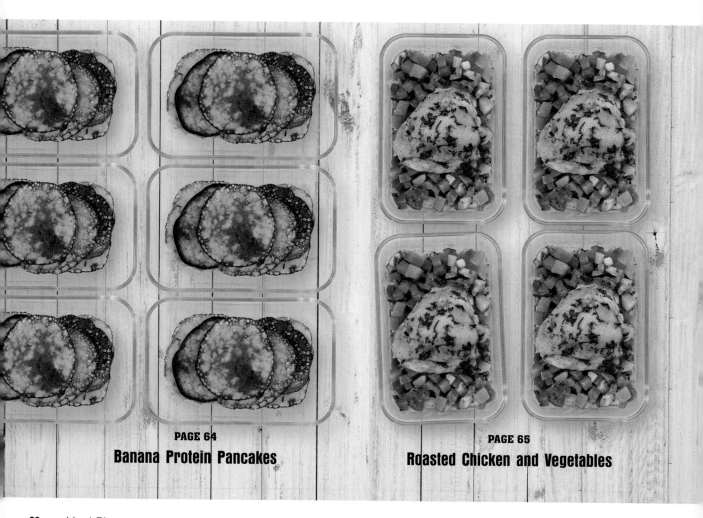

PAGE 64
Banana Protein Pancakes

PAGE 65
Roasted Chicken and Vegetables

Awesome Arrowroot

Arrowroot flour is made from the starch of tropical tubers. It has anti-inflammatory properties and is easy to digest. It's great for thickening sauces and coating meats.

Safe Spiralizing

If using a hand-held spiralizer to make **zucchini noodles,** use a fork to hold the end of the zucchini in place and keep your fingers away from the blades.

SOMETHING TO MUNCH ON

- Spread apple slices with natural peanut butter for a sweet burst of energy.

- Try roasted pumpkin seeds, or make your own roasted butternut squash seeds.

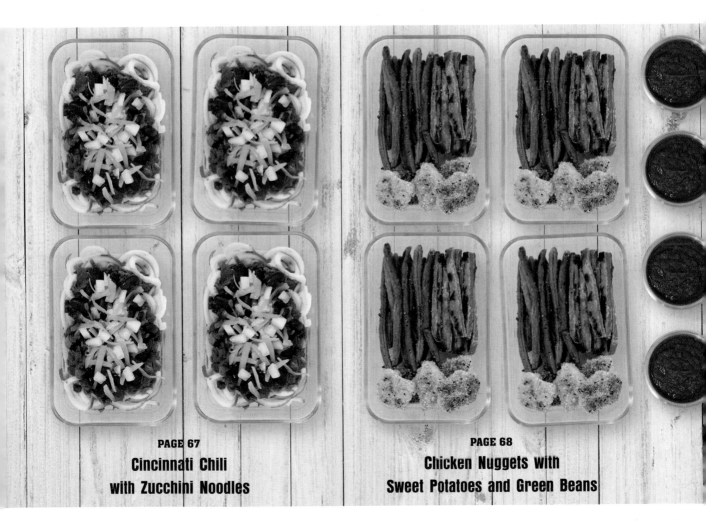

PAGE 67
Cincinnati Chili with Zucchini Noodles

PAGE 68
Chicken Nuggets with Sweet Potatoes and Green Beans

Prep Day Action Plan

EQUIPMENT
Chef's knife
Cutting board
Mixing bowls
Shallow bowls (2)
Measuring cups
Measuring spoons
Large non-stick sauté pan with lid
Large non-stick frying pan
Baking sheets (2)
Aluminum foil
Spiralizer
Blender
Colander or mesh sieve
Meal prep containers (18)
Food scale (optional)

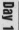 Cozy Comfort Food
shopping list, p146

1 Preheat the oven to 400°F (200°C). Squeeze a lemon into a large bowl and begin marinating the chicken for the **roasted chicken and vegetables (p65, step 1).**

2 While the chicken marinates, prepare the vegetables.
1 medium butternut squash, deseeded, peeled, and cubed
2 medium zucchini squash, cut into chunks
1 medium sweet potatoes (unpeeled), cut into chunks
4 garlic cloves, papery skins removed
➡ Place in a large bowl.

3 Line a baking sheet with foil and continue preparing the roasted **chicken and vegetables (p65, steps 2–3).** Put the tray in the oven and set a timer for 45 minutes.

4 While the chicken and vegetables are roasting, prepare ingredients for the chili.

1 medium yellow onion, diced
4 garlic cloves, minced
➡ Place in a medium bowl.

4 medium zucchini squash, spiralized
➡ Place in a large bowl.

5 Measure spices for the chili. Combine 1 tsp ground cumin, 1 tsp cinnamon, ¼ tsp allspice, ⅛ tsp cayenne pepper, and 1 tbsp raw cacao powder in a small bowl.

Week at a Glance

Day 1
Breakfast Banana Protein Pancakes
Lunch Cincinnati Chili
Dinner Roasted Chicken and Vegetables

Day 2
Breakfast Banana Protein Pancakes
Lunch Chicken Nuggets
Dinner Cincinnati Chili

Day 3
Breakfast Banana Protein Pancakes
Lunch Roasted Chicken and Vegetables
Dinner Chicken Nuggets

6 Begin preparing the **chili (p67, steps 1–3).** Once the chili is simmering, check the chicken and vegetables. When the timer goes off, remove from the oven and set aside to cool before assembling your meals.

7 Finish preparing the zucchini noodles for the **chili (p67, steps 4–6).** Then wash and prepare ingredients for the chicken nuggets and ketchup.

For the chicken nuggets:
2 sweet potatoes, cut into fries
➡ Place in a medium bowl.

For the ketchup:
½ medium yellow onion, diced
4 garlic cloves, minced
➡ Place in a small bowl.

8 Make the sweet potatoes and green beans for the **chicken nuggets (p68, steps 1–4).** While the green beans are in the oven, assemble the Cincinnati chili and roasted chicken meals.

9 Cut 1¼lb (600g) chicken breast into nugget-size pieces. Prepare the **chicken nuggets (p68, steps 5–6).** Then make the **ketchup (p17, all steps)** and assemble the chicken nugget meals.

10 Make the **banana pancakes (p64, all steps).** Make as many batches as you need for the week.

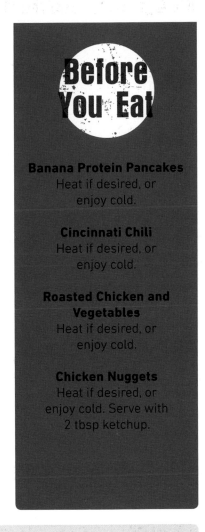

Before You Eat

Banana Protein Pancakes
Heat if desired, or enjoy cold.

Cincinnati Chili
Heat if desired, or enjoy cold.

Roasted Chicken and Vegetables
Heat if desired, or enjoy cold.

Chicken Nuggets
Heat if desired, or enjoy cold. Serve with 2 tbsp ketchup.

Day 4
Breakfast Banana Protein Pancakes
Lunch Cincinnati Chili
Dinner Roasted Chicken and Vegetables

Day 5
Breakfast Banana Protein Pancakes
Lunch Chicken Nuggets
Dinner Cincinnati Chili

Day 6
Breakfast Banana Protein Pancakes
Lunch Roasted Chicken and Vegetables
Dinner Chicken Nuggets

This recipe makes one serving of pancakes at a time, so prepare as many or as few batches as you need for the week.

Banana Protein Pancakes

PREP TIME 12 minutes   **COOK TIME** 30 minutes   **MAKES** 6 servings   **SERVING SIZE** 6 pancakes

NUTRITION PER SERVING Protein 32g / Carbohydrates 30g / Fiber 3g / Sugars 15g / Fat 25g / Calories 473

12 eggs

6 bananas

12 tbsp undenatured whey protein

6 tbsp coconut oil

1 To make one serving of pancakes, combine 2 eggs, 1 banana, and 2 tbsp whey protein in a blender and blend until well combined.

2 In a large, non-stick frying pan, melt ½ tbsp coconut oil over high heat, then reduce heat to medium. Using about half of the batter, form 3 pancakes. Cook for 1 minute, until pancakes appear slightly dry and set on top.

3 Flip the pancakes and cook for 1 minute more. Pancakes should be cooked through and golden brown on both sides. Transfer the cooked pancakes to a meal prep container. Make another 3 pancakes with the remaining batter and add to the container.

4 To finish your meal prep for the week, repeat steps 1 to 3 to make 5 more servings of pancakes.

TIP
Flavored protein powders taste great in these pancakes. Try strawberry, chocolate, or vanilla.

Roasted chicken is comfort food at its best. As the chicken cooks, its juices infuse the vegetables with savory flavor.

Roasted Chicken and Vegetables

PREP TIME 20 minutes   **COOK TIME** 45 minutes   **MAKES** 4 servings   **SERVING SIZE** 1 assembled meal

NUTRITION PER SERVING Protein 35g / Carbohydrates 38g / Fiber 7g / Sugars 16g / Fat 31g / Calories 571

6 tbsp olive oil

Juice of 1 lemon

2 tbsp chopped fresh rosemary

4 skin-on, bone-in chicken thighs, about 1¼lb (600g) in total

Salt and freshly ground black pepper

1 medium butternut squash, cubed, about 2lb (1kg) in total

2 medium zucchini squash, cut into chunks, about 14oz (400g) in total

1 medium sweet potato, cut into chunks, about 10½oz (300g) in total

4 garlic cloves, whole (optional)

1 Preheat oven to 400°F (200°C). In a large bowl, stir together 2 tbsp olive oil, lemon juice, and 1 tbsp rosemary. Add the chicken thighs, season with salt and pepper, and toss well to coat. Refrigerate for 15 to 20 minutes to marinate.
➡ *Return to Prep Day Action Plan while chicken marinates.*

2 In a large bowl, combine the butternut squash, zucchini, sweet potatoes, and garlic cloves, if using. Season with salt and pepper and add the remaining 4 tbsp olive oil and remaining 1 tbsp fresh rosemary. Toss to coat.

3 Spread the vegetables on a foil-lined baking sheet. Take the chicken out of the refrigerator and arrange on top of the vegetables, drizzling the leftover marinade over top. Place in the oven for 45 minutes, until chicken skin is browned and crisp and meat is cooked through.
➡ *Return to Prep Day Action Plan while chicken roasts.*

4 To assemble the meals, divide the vegetables evenly among 4 containers and add 1 chicken thigh to each container.

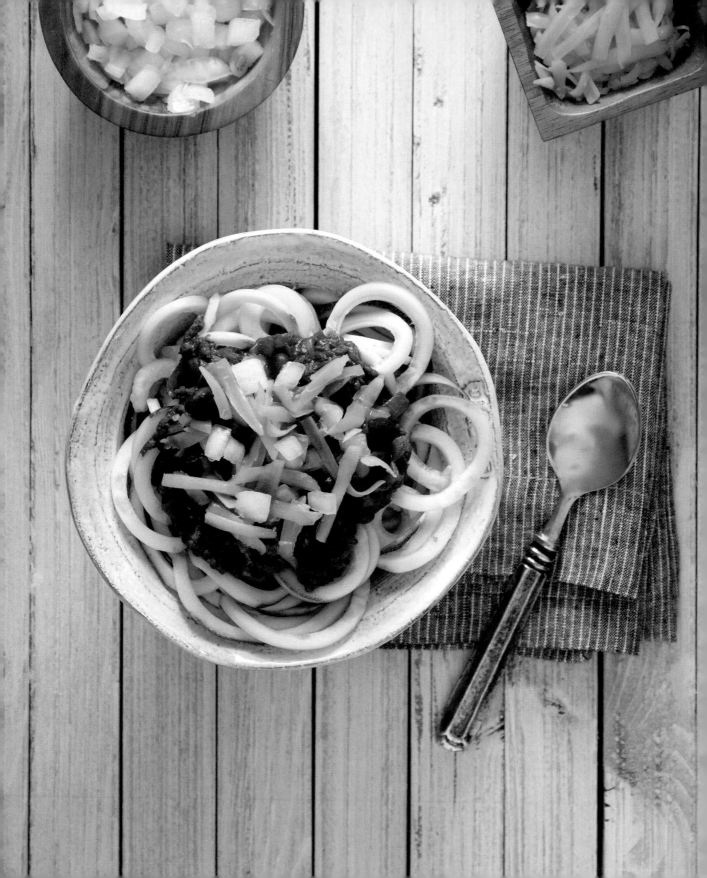

Hearty beef and bean chili tops zucchini noodles instead of traditional spaghetti in this healthy twist on a regional classic.

Cincinnati Chili
with Zucchini Noodles

PREP TIME 20 minutes   **COOK TIME** 45 minutes   **MAKES** 4 servings   **SERVING SIZE** 1 assembled meal

NUTRITION PER SERVING Protein 45g / Carbohydrates 40g / Fiber 15g / Sugars 13g / Fat 28g / Calories 592

FOR CHILI

1 tbsp olive oil

4 garlic cloves, minced

1 medium yellow onion, diced

2 tbsp tomato paste

1lb (450g) ground beef

4 cups beef broth

1 cup tomato purée

1 tbsp apple cider vinegar

1 tbsp chili powder

1 tsp ground cumin

1 tsp cinnamon

1/4 tsp allspice

1/8 tsp cayenne pepper

1 tbsp raw cacao powder

15oz (425g) can kidney beans, drained and rinsed

1/2 cup shredded cheddar cheese (optional)

FOR ZUCCHINI NOODLES

1 tbsp olive oil

4 garlic cloves, minced

4 medium zucchini squash, spiralized, about 1¾lb (800g) in total

1 To make the chili, heat olive oil in a large, non-stick pan over medium heat. Add the garlic and onion and cook for 2 minutes.

2 Add the tomato paste and ground beef, using a wooden spoon to break up the meat. Cook until the meat is browned, about 3 minutes.

3 Add the beef broth, tomato purée, apple cider vinegar, chili powder, cumin, cinnamon, allspice, cayenne pepper, and cacao powder. Stir until well combined. Bring to a boil, then reduce the heat and simmer for 30 minutes, stirring occasionally.
➡ *Return to Prep Day Action Plan.*

4 To make the zucchini noodles, heat olive oil in a large, non-stick sauté pan over high heat. Add garlic and sauté for 1 minute. Add the spiralized zucchini, cover, and cook for 2 minutes. Remove the lid and toss the zucchini noodles with tongs, then replace the lid and cook for another 3 to 4 minutes, until the zucchini begins to soften.

5 Transfer the zucchini noodles to a colander and drain. Spread the drained noodles on a baking sheet lined with paper towel, and press with additional paper towel to absorb moisture.

6 To assemble the meals, divide the zucchini noodles evenly among 4 containers. Top the noodles with the chili and kidney beans, and sprinkle each portion with 2 tbsp shredded cheddar cheese, if using.

A cornmeal crust keeps these chicken nuggets moist and tender. They freeze well, so make extra to keep on hand.

Chicken Nuggets
with Sweet Potatoes and Green Beans

PREP TIME 20 minutes   **COOK TIME** 50 minutes   **MAKES** 4 servings   **SERVING SIZE** 1 assembled meal

NUTRITION PER SERVING Protein 38g / Carbohydrates 38g / Fiber 6g / Sugars 6g / Fat 23g / Calories 508

FOR VEGETABLES

2 medium sweet potatoes, about 1lb (500g) total, sliced into fries

2 tbsp arrowroot flour

2 tbsp olive oil

Salt and freshly ground black pepper

8oz (250g) green beans, trimmed

FOR CHICKEN NUGGETS

½ cup coarsely ground cornmeal or polenta

¼ cup arrowroot flour

½ tsp salt

¼ tsp freshly ground black pepper

1 egg

1¼ lb (600g) skinless, boneless chicken breast, cut into nugget-sized pieces

4 tbsp olive oil

¼ cup **Ketchup** (see p17), to serve

1 Preheat the oven to 450°F (230°C) and line a baking sheet with parchment paper. In a large bowl, toss sweet potatoes with 1 tbsp arrowroot flour to coat. Drizzle with 1 tbsp olive oil and season with salt and pepper. Toss together and spread on the baking sheet. Bake for 15 minutes.

2 In the same bowl, toss the green beans with remaining 1 tbsp arrowroot flour. Drizzle with remaining 1 tbsp olive oil and season with salt and pepper. Set aside.

3 Remove the potatoes from the oven, turn each one, and return to the oven for 15 minutes, until cooked through. Divide the potatoes evenly among 4 meal prep containers.

4 Spread the green beans on the same baking sheet and bake for 10 minutes. Add to meal prep containers with sweet potatoes.
➡ *Return to Prep Day Action Plan while green beans roast.*

5 To make the chicken nuggets, whisk together the cornmeal, arrowroot flour, salt, and pepper in a shallow bowl. In a separate shallow bowl, whisk the egg. Working in batches, coat the raw chicken pieces with the egg wash, then transfer them to the cornmeal mixture and toss to coat.

6 In a large, non-stick sauté pan, heat 2 tbsp olive oil. Add half of the chicken to the hot pan and cook for 3 to 4 minutes on each side until golden brown. Repeat with the remaining chicken.

7 To assemble the meals, divide the chicken evenly among the 4 containers. Serve each meal with 2 tbsp ketchup.

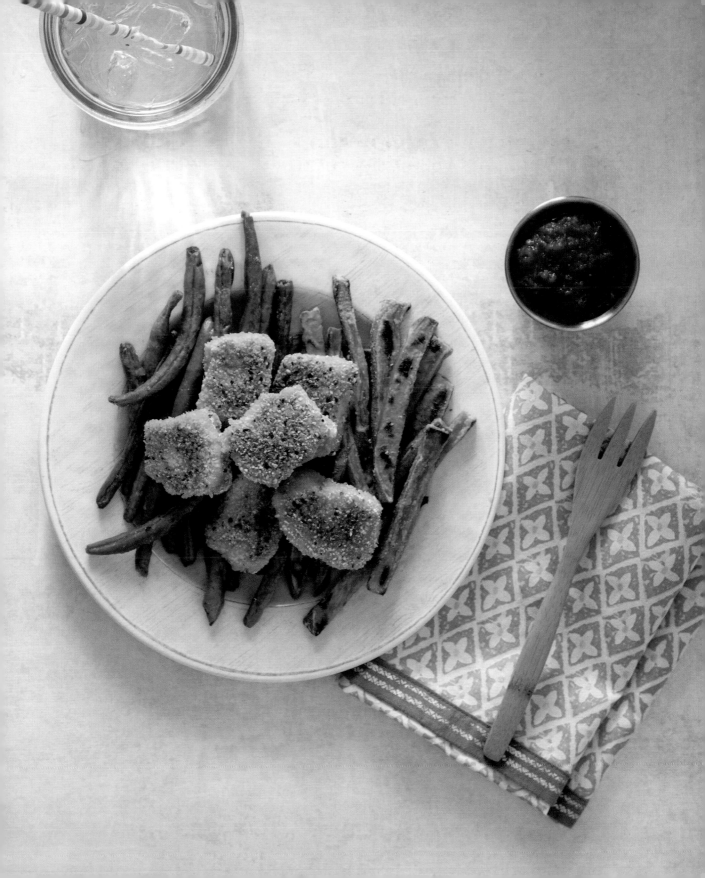

Mediterranean Meals

These meals draw on the classic flavors of Italy and Greece, with garlic, lemon, and herbs seasoning each dish. Light but satisfying, these recipes feature plenty of fresh vegetables and lean protein to keep you full.

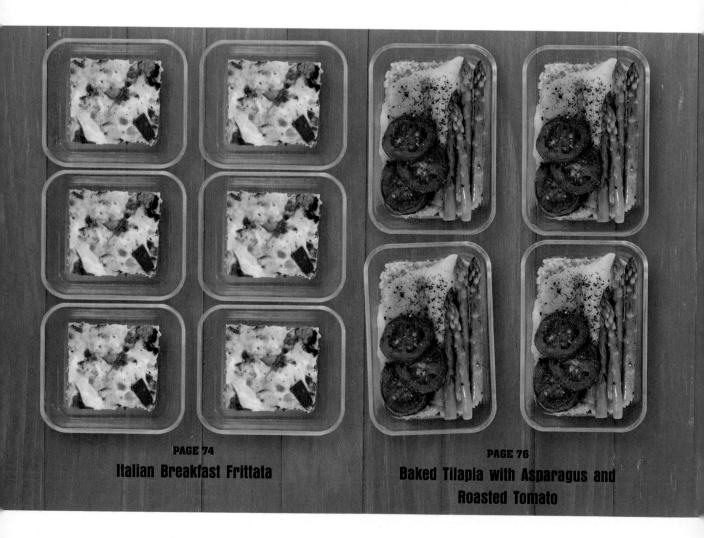

PAGE 74
Italian Breakfast Frittata

PAGE 76
Baked Tilapia with Asparagus and Roasted Tomato

Flaxseed Oil

The Greek salad gets an omega-3 boost from **flaxseed oil**. Flaxseed oil is perfect for dressings, but is unstable at high temperatures and not suitable for cooking.

Vegetarian Swap

Leave out the **sausage** and add chopped **mushrooms** to the **Italian Breakfast Frittata** for a meat-free morning.

SOMETHING TO MUNCH ON

- Cucumber slices with tzatziki are a quick and low-carb snack.

- Toss chickpeas with olive oil and seasonings and roast at 425°F (218°C) for 20 minutes for a protein-packed, crispy snack.

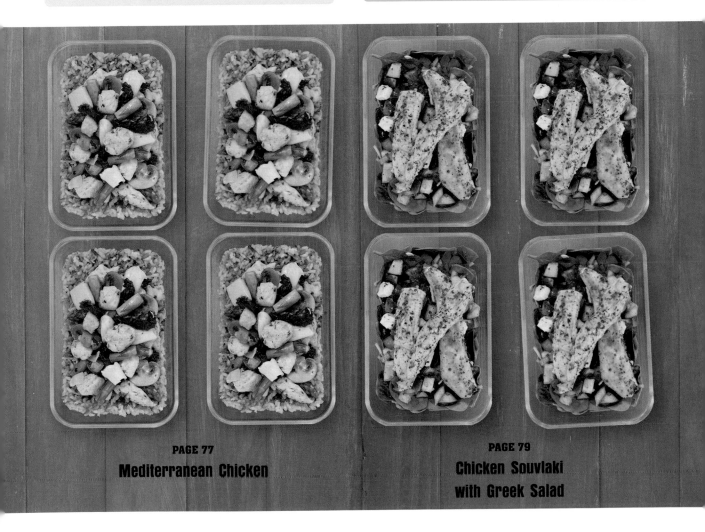

PAGE 77
Mediterranean Chicken

PAGE 79
Chicken Souvlaki with Greek Salad

Prep Day Action Plan

EQUIPMENT

Chef's knife

Cutting board

Mixing bowls

Measuring cups

Measuring spoons

Large non-stick sauté pan

Medium saucepans (2)

9 x 13in (23 x 33cm) baking dish

Baking sheets (2)

Aluminum foil

Spatula

Whisk

Lemon juicer

Kitchen shears

Mesh sieve

Meal prep containers (18)

Food scale (optional)

 Mediterranean Meals shopping list, p147

1 Wash and prepare **frittata** ingredients:
1 small yellow onion, diced
➡ Place in small bowl.

1 medium zucchini, diced
1 red bell pepper, diced
➡ Place in a medium bowl.

3 cups kale, chopped
➡ Place in a medium bowl.

2 Grate 8oz (225g) mozzarella and remove sausage casings. Begin preparing **frittata (p74, steps 1–5).** Set a timer for 25 minutes.

3 While the frittata bakes, prepare rice according to package directions. You will need about ¾ cup uncooked brown rice to yield 2 cups cooked.

4 In another saucepan, prepare quinoa according to package directions. You will need about ½ cup uncooked quinoa to yield 2 cups cooked.

5 Slice 4 Roma tomatoes and begin preparing the **baked tilapia (p76, steps 1–2).** Check the rice and quinoa and remove from heat when cooked.

6 When timer goes off, remove the frittata from the oven and set aside to cool before portioning into containers. Put fish and tomatoes in the oven and set a timer for 12 minutes.

Week at a Glance

Day 1
Breakfast Italian Breakfast Frittata
Lunch Baked Tilapia
Dinner Chicken Souvlaki

Day 2
Breakfast Italian Breakfast Frittata
Lunch Mediterranean Chicken
Dinner Baked Tilapia

Day 3
Breakfast Italian Breakfast Frittata
Lunch Baked Tilapia
Dinner Chicken Souvlaki

7 While fish bakes, slice 1 yellow onion and trim 1 bunch asparagus. Prepare the vegetables for the **baked tilapia (p76, step 3).** When the timer goes off, assemble the meals.

8 Wipe out your pan. Prepare ingredients for the Mediterranean chicken and chicken souvlaki.

For the Mediterranean chicken:
1 bunch asparagus, trimmed and diced
8oz mushrooms, sliced
➡ Place in medium bowl.

½ cup sundried tomatoes, diced
8 canned artichokes, diced
➡ Place in small bowl.

For the chicken souvlaki:
1 medium cucumber, diced
2 medium tomatoes, diced
8oz (225g) feta cheese, cubed
½ small red onion, diced
➡ Place in a medium bowl.

9 Trim and slice 1⅓lb (600g) chicken breast into strips. Prepare the **Mediterranean chicken (p77, all steps).**

10 Trim and slice 1⅓lb (600g) chicken breast into strips. Prepare the **chicken souvlaki (p79, all steps).**

Before You Eat

Italian Breakfast Frittata
Enjoy cold or briefly heat until warm.

Baked Tilapia
Heat briefly to warm. Extended heating will make fish rubbery.

Mediterranean Chicken
Heat if desired, or enjoy cold.

Chicken Souvlaki
Enjoy cold. Top with 2 tbsp Greek yogurt before serving.

Day 4
Breakfast Italian Breakfast Frittata
Lunch Mediterranean Chicken
Dinner Baked Tilapia

Day 5
Breakfast Italian Breakfast Frittata
Lunch Chicken Souvlaki
Dinner Mediterranean Chicken

Day 6
Breakfast Italian Breakfast Frittata
Lunch Mediterranean Chicken
Dinner Chicken Souvlaki

This savory egg casserole is packed with sausage, cheese, and tons of veggies for a hearty morning meal.

Italian Breakfast Frittata

PREP TIME 15 minutes **COOK TIME** 35 minutes **MAKES** 6 servings **SERVING SIZE** ⅙ of pan

NUTRITION PER SERVING Protein 27g / Carbohydrates 12g / Fiber 3g / Sugars 5g / Fat 33g / Calories 453

4 tbsp olive oil

8oz (225g) sweet or spicy Italian sausage, casings removed

1 small yellow onion, diced, about 4½oz (125g) in total

1 red bell pepper, diced, about 7oz (200g) in total

1 medium zucchini squash, diced, about 7oz (200g) in total

3 cups chopped kale

Handful of fresh basil leaves, roughly torn

12 eggs

½ cup half and half

8oz (225g) full-fat mozzarella cheese, grated

1 tsp dried Italian seasoning

Salt and freshly ground black pepper

1 Preheat the oven to 375°F (190°C) and grease a 9 x 13in (23 x 33cm) baking dish with 2 tbsp olive oil. In a large, non-stick sauté pan, heat 1 tbsp olive oil over medium heat. Add the sausage and stir, using a spatula to break up the meat. Once the sausage starts to brown, cook for 3 to 4 minutes. Spread the cooked sausage evenly in the prepared baking dish.

2 To the same pan, heat remaining 1 tbsp olive oil over medium heat. Add the onion and sauté for 2 to 3 minutes. Add the bell pepper and zucchini and cook for another 3 to 4 minutes, stirring occasionally, until the vegetables have softened. Add the kale and stir until wilted, about 1 minute.

3 Evenly distribute the vegetables over the sausage in the baking dish. Sprinkle the torn basil over top.

4 In a large bowl, whisk the eggs until whites and yolks are well combined. Whisk in the half and half, mozzarella, and Italian seasoning, and season with salt and pepper.

5 Pour the egg mixture evenly over the sausage and vegetables and bake for 25 minutes, or until the eggs are set and the top is beginning to brown.
➡ *Return to Prep Day Action Plan while frittata bakes.*

6 To assemble the meals, cut the frittata into 6 pieces and place in meal prep containers.

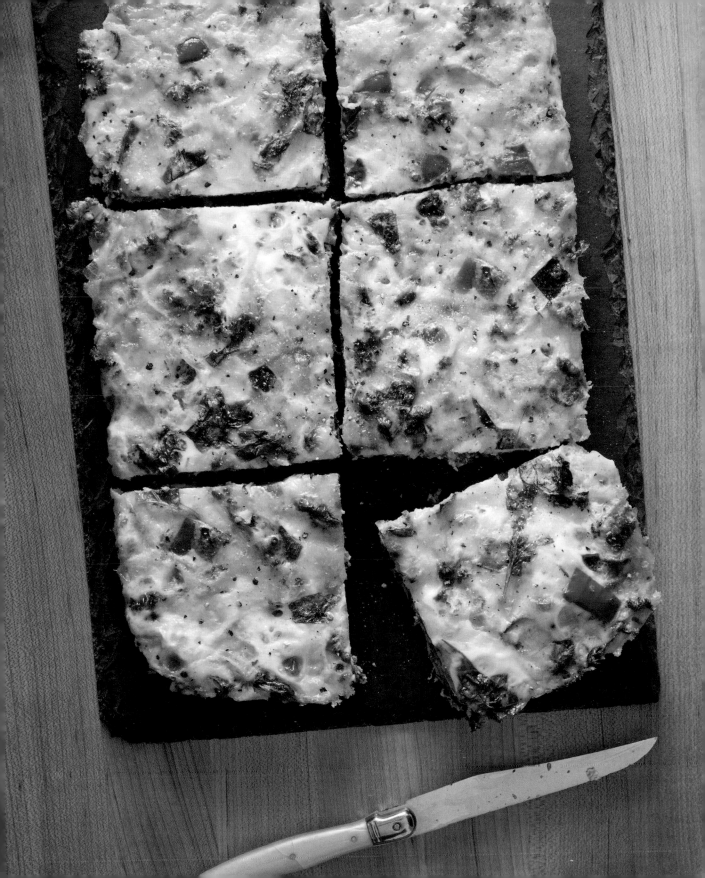

Roasting tomatoes deepens their flavor, making them less tart and perfect for pairing with mild tilapia and asparagus.

Baked Tilapia
with Asparagus and Roasted Tomatoes

PREP TIME 10 minutes   **COOK TIME** 20 minutes   **MAKES** 4 servings   **SERVING SIZE** 1 assembled meal

NUTRITION PER SERVING Protein 27g / Carbohydrates 29g / Fiber 6g / Sugars 5g / Fat 25g / Calories 449

4 tilapia fillets, each about 4oz (125g)

6 tbsp olive oil

2 tbsp freshly squeezed lemon juice (about 1 large lemon)

Salt and freshly ground black pepper

2 tbsp dried Italian seasoning

4 Roma tomatoes, cut into thirds, about 14oz (400g) in total

1 small yellow onion, thinly sliced, about 5oz (150g) in total

1 bunch asparagus, trimmed, about 14oz (400g) in total

2 cups cooked quinoa

1 Preheat the oven to 375°F (190°C) and line 2 baking sheets with foil. Arrange the fish on one baking sheet and drizzle with 2 tbsp olive oil and 1 tbsp lemon juice. Sprinkle with salt, pepper, and ½ tbsp Italian seasoning, then flip and repeat to season the opposite side.

2 On the other baking sheet, arrange the tomato slices and drizzle with 2 tbsp olive oil. Sprinkle with salt, pepper, and remaining 1 tbsp Italian seasoning. Put both trays in the oven, fish on top rack, and bake for 12 to 15 minutes, or until the fish flakes easily with a fork.
➡ *Return to Prep Day Action Plan while tomatoes and fish bake.*

3 In a large non-stick pan, heat remaining 2 tbsp olive oil over medium-high heat. Add the onion and cook for 2 to 3 minutes. Spread the asparagus over the onion and sprinkle with salt and pepper. Cover and cook over medium heat for 5 to 6 minutes. Stir in the remaining 1 tbsp lemon juice and remove from heat.

4 To assemble the meals, add ½ cup cooked quinoa to each of 4 containers. Divide the tomatoes, asparagus, and onions evenly among the containers, and add 1 piece of fish to each.

Artichokes, sundried tomatoes, and fresh thyme flavor this medley of chicken and vegetables, served on a bed of rice.

Mediterranean Chicken

PREP TIME 10 minutes   **COOK TIME** 10 minutes   **MAKES** 4 servings   **SERVING SIZE** 1 assembled meal

NUTRITION PER SERVING Protein 43g / Carbohydrates 37g / Fiber 9g / Sugars 6g / Fat 19g / Calories 491

4 tbsp olive oil

1⅓lb (600g) skinless, boneless chicken breast, diced

Salt and freshly ground black pepper

1 tbsp chopped fresh thyme

1 bunch asparagus, trimmed and cut into bite-size pieces, about 14oz (400g) in total

8oz (225g) button mushrooms, sliced

½ cup oil-packed sundried tomatoes, diced

8 canned artichoke hearts, about 4oz (120g) total, cut into bite-size pieces

2 cups cooked brown rice

1 In a large wok, heat 2 tbsp olive oil over medium-high heat. Add the chicken and season with salt and pepper. Cook, stirring occasionally, for 3 to 4 minutes, or until the chicken is white on all sides and the juices run clear. Once the chicken is fully cooked, transfer to a bowl and set aside.

2 To the same pan, add the remaining 2 tbsp olive oil and thyme. Cook over medium heat for 1 minute, then add the asparagus and mushrooms. Cook for 3 minutes more, stirring occasionally, or until the mushrooms begin to brown.

3 Add the sundried tomatoes and artichokes and cook for 3 minutes more, stirring occasionally. Season salt and pepper. Add the cooked chicken to the pan and stir. Remove from heat.

4 To assemble the meals, add ½ cup cooked rice to each of 4 containers. Divide the chicken and vegetables evenly among the containers.

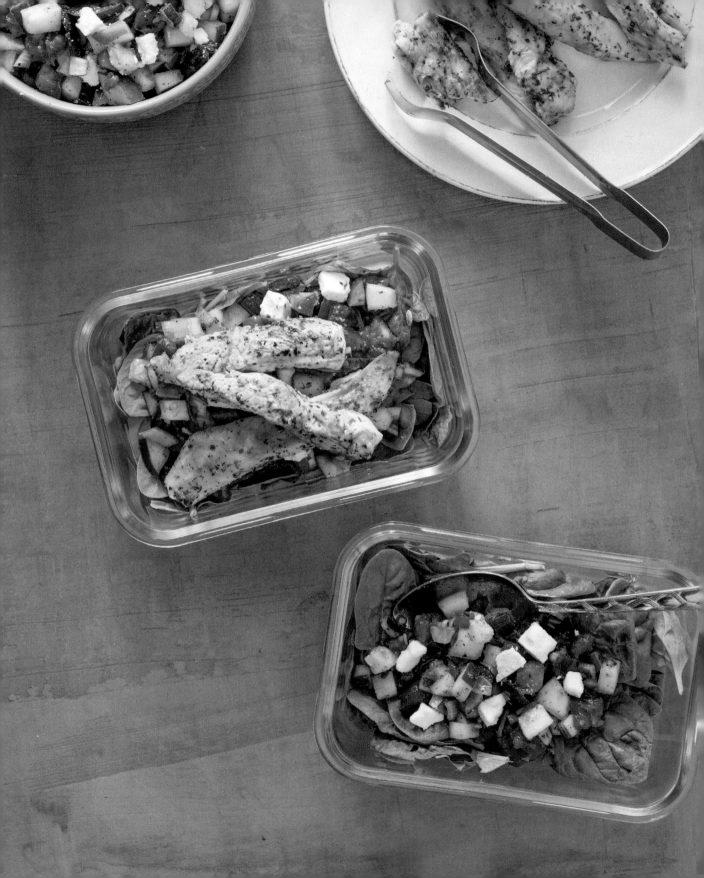

Bursting with Greek flavors, chicken is marinated in lemon, garlic, and oregano and served with a crisp cucumber salad.

Chicken Souvlaki
with Greek Salad

PREP TIME 15 minutes   **COOK TIME** 10 minutes   **MAKES** 4 servings   **SERVING SIZE** 1 assembled meal

NUTRITION PER SERVING Protein 48g / Carbohydrates 13g / Fiber 2g / Sugars 5g / Fat 37g / Calories 577

4 garlic cloves, minced

Juice of 2 lemons

4 tbsp olive oil

3 tbsp dried oregano

¼ tsp salt

¼ tsp freshly ground black pepper

1⅓lb (600g) skinless, boneless chicken breast, cut into strips

1 medium cucumber, diced

2 medium tomatoes, diced, about 14oz (400g) in total

8oz (225g) feta cheese, cubed

½ small red onion, diced, about 3½oz (100g) in total

20 pitted Kalamata olives, about 2oz (60g) total, halved

2 tbsp flaxseed oil

2 cups baby spinach

½ cup full-fat Greek yogurt, to serve

1 In a large bowl, whisk together the garlic, lemon juice, 3 tbsp olive oil, 2 tbsp oregano, salt, and pepper. Add the chicken strips and mix together.

2 In a large non-stick sauté pan, heat remaining 1 tbsp olive oil over high heat. Add the chicken and cook for 2 to 3 minutes on each side, until it is cooked through and the juices run clear. Set aside to cool.

3 In a medium bowl, toss the cucumber, tomatoes, feta cheese, red onion, and olives with the flaxseed oil and remaining 1 tbsp dried oregano. Add salt and pepper to taste.

4 To assemble the meals, place a small handful of baby spinach in each of 4 containers. Add a scoop of salad to each, and divide the chicken evenly among the containers. To serve, top each meal with 2 tbsp Greek yogurt.

TIP
For more authentic flavor, put the chicken on skewers and cook on the grill.

Diner Delights

Bring your favorite diner food into your kitchen with this week's meals. Craving pancakes, burgers, or fish and chips? These recipes will leaving you feeling fully satisfied, but not heavy, with reasonable portion sizes so you don't overeat.

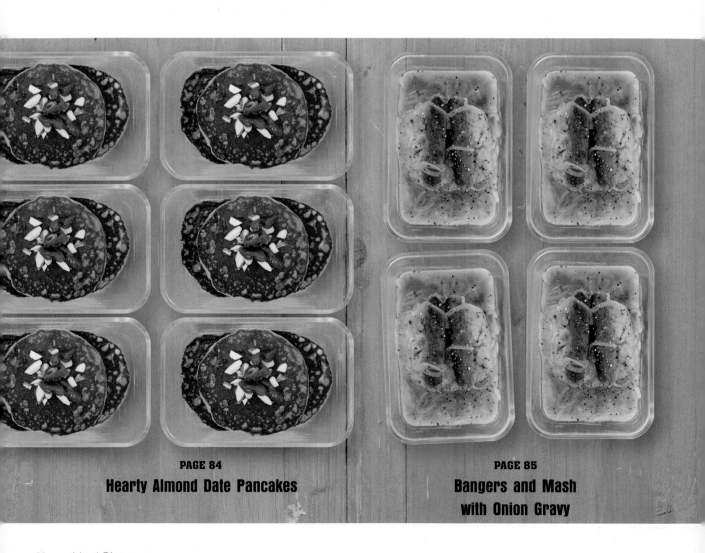

PAGE 84
Hearty Almond Date Pancakes

PAGE 85
**Bangers and Mash
with Onion Gravy**

Russet Potatoes

Regular **potatoes** get a bad rap, but they have fewer carbs and less sugar than sweet potatoes, as well as different nurients, so it's good to get a healthy mix of both in your diet.

Sausage Swap

If you don't eat pork, use **chicken sausage** for the **Bangers and Mash**, or try a meatless variety.

SOMETHING TO MUNCH ON

- Prepare 2oz (55g) bags of nuts to get the benefit of healthy fats without overeating.

- A hardboiled egg is filling and has 6 grams of protein, 5 grams of fat, and less than 1 gram of carbs.

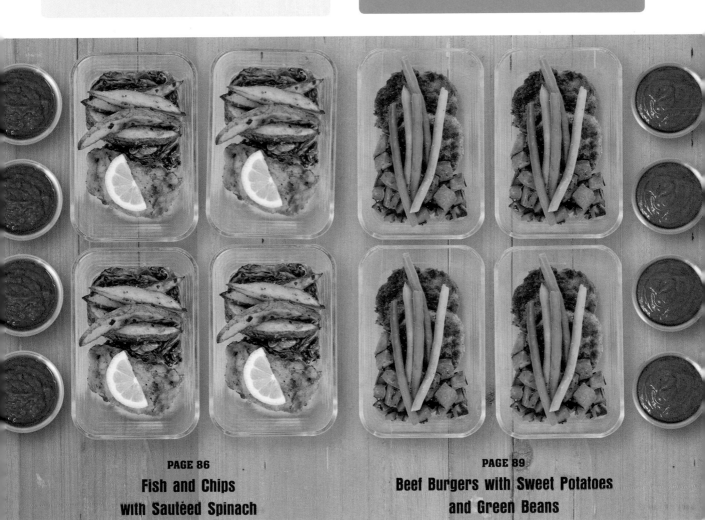

PAGE 86

Fish and Chips with Sautéed Spinach

PAGE 89

Beef Burgers with Sweet Potatoes and Green Beans

Prep Day Action Plan

EQUIPMENT

Chef's knife

Cutting board

Mixing bowls

Measuring cups

Measuring spoons

Large, non-stick sauté pan with lid

Pot with steamer insert

Baking sheets (2)

Aluminum foil or parchment paper

Whisk

Spatula

Food processor

Meal prep containers (18)

Food scale (optional)

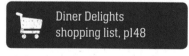

 Diner Delights
shopping list, p148

1 Preheat the oven to 450°F (230°C) and line 2 baking sheets with foil or parchment paper. Prepare the following ingredients.

For the beef burgers:
2 sweet potatoes, diced
1 tbsp chopped fresh thyme
➡ Place in medium bowl.
14oz (400g) green beans, trimmed
➡ Place in steamer insert.

For the fish and chips:
2 russet potatoes, cut into fries
3 garlic cloves, minced
➡ Place in medium bowl.

For the ketchup:
½ medium yellow onion, diced
4 garlic cloves, minced
➡ Place in a small bowl.

For the bangers and mash:
2 heads cauliflower, cut into florets
➡ Place in a medium bowl.

2 Prepare the sweet potatoes for the **beef burgers (p89, step 1)** and the potatoes for the **fish and chips (p86, step 1).** Put both baking sheets in the oven and set a timer for 25 minutes.

Week at a Glance

 Day 1

Breakfast Hearty Almond Date Pancakes

Lunch Fish and Chips

Dinner Bangers and Mash

Day 2

Breakfast Hearty Almond Date Pancakes

Lunch Beef Burgers

Dinner Fish and Chips

 Day 3

Breakfast Hearty Almond Date Pancakes

Lunch Fish and Chips

Dinner Bangers and Mash

3 While the potatoes bake, set up the steamer and steam the green beans for the **beef burgers (p89, step 2).**

4 While the green beans steam, begin cooking the **pancakes (p84, all steps).** If the green beans finish cooking before you're finished making the pancakes, remove from heat and set aside.

5 When the timer for the potatoes goes off, divide the fries evenly among 4 containers and divide the diced sweet potatoes evenly among another 4 containers. When the green beans are cooked, add them to the containers with the sweet potato.

6 Rinse out the steamer pot and steam the cauliflower for the **bangers and mash (p85, step 1).**

7 Slice 1 small onion and finish preparing the **bangers and mash (p85, steps 2–7)**.

8 Batter and cook the cod and spinach for the **fish and chips (p86, steps 2–5)** and add to the containers with the fries. Top with lemon slices and refrigerate the meals.

9 Wipe out your pan and prepare the **beef burgers (p89, steps 3–5).** Add the burgers to the containers with the green beans and sweet potatoes.

10 Make **BBQ Sauce (p16, all steps).** Add 2 tbsp to each burger patty. Make the **Ketchup (p17, all steps).** Refrigerate until ready to serve with fish and chips.

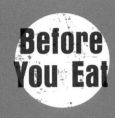

Before You Eat

Hearty Almond and Date Pancakes
Briefly warm if desired, or enjoy cold.

Fish and Chips
Heat if desired, or enjoy cold. Serve with 2 tbsp ketchup.

Bangers and Mash
Heat if desired, or enjoy cold.

Beef Burgers
Heat if desired, or enjoy cold. Add lettuce, tomato, and onion after heating, if using.

Day 4
Breakfast Hearty Almond Date Pancakes
Lunch Beef Burgers
Dinner Fish and Chips

Day 5
Breakfast Hearty Almond Date Pancakes
Lunch Bangers and Mash
Dinner Beef Burgers

Day 6
Breakfast Hearty Almond Date Pancakes
Lunch Beef Burgers
Dinner Bangers and Mash

You won't need syrup for these gluten-free pancakes. Dates and bananas give them a natural sweetness and cake-like texture.

Hearty Almond Date Pancakes

PREP TIME 10 minutes   **COOK TIME** 15 minutes   **MAKES** 6 servings   **SERVING SIZE** 2 to 3 pancakes, 4in (10cm) across

NUTRITION PER SERVING Protein 25g / Carbohydrates 31g / Fiber 5g / Sugars 17g / Fat 32g / Calories 512

½ cup whole pitted dates, tightly packed, about 3½oz (100g) in total

1½ cups whole, raw almonds

3 bananas, cut into chunks

½ cup coconut oil, melted, plus extra for frying

1½ cups undenatured whey protein

1 tbsp cinnamon

1 Place dates in a small bowl and add boiling water to cover. Let soak for 5 minutes.

2 In a food processor, process almonds until they reach a finely ground, flour-like consistency. Add bananas and ½ cup coconut oil and process until smooth and well combined.

3 Drain the dates and add them to the food processor, along with whey protein and cinnamon. Process until well combined.

4 In a large, non-stick frying pan, melt 2 tsp coconut oil over medium heat. Cook the pancakes in batches, using a ¼-cup measure to scoop the batter in the hot pan. Cook for 2 to 3 minutes, until the pancakes look dry around the edges, then carefully flip and cook the opposite side for another 2 to 3 minutes. Transfer the cooked pancakes to a cooling rack and continue making pancakes until batter is gone.

5 Divide the pancakes evenly among 6 airtight containers and top with additional chopped dates and almonds, if desired.

TIP

Instead of processing raw almonds in step 2, you can use 1½ cups almond flour.

The classic pairing of sausage and mashed potatoes gets a low-carb update with mashed cauliflower and onion gravy.

Bangers and Mash
with Onion Gravy

PREP TIME 10 minutes   **COOK TIME** 20 minutes   **MAKES** 4 servings   **SERVING SIZE** 1 assembled meal

NUTRITION PER SERVING Protein 30g / Carbohydrates 23g / Fiber 8g / Sugars 9g / Fat 41g / Calories 560

2 heads cauliflower, cut into small pieces, about 2lb (1kg) in total

2 tbsp olive oil

1 medium yellow onion, sliced

8 pork sausages, about 2½oz (75g) each

2 tbsp arrowroot flour

2 cups cold water

2 tbsp butter

2 garlic cloves, minced

1 tbsp dried Italian seasoning

¼ tsp ground nutmeg

¼ tsp salt

¼ tsp freshly ground black pepper

1 In a pot with a steamer insert, steam the cauliflower for 12 to 15 minutes, or until easily pierced with a fork. Set aside.

2 In a large non-stick pan, heat olive oil over medium-high heat. Add the onion and cook until beginning to soften, about 3 minutes. Push the onions to the side and add sausages. Cook for 2 to 3 minutes, then turn the sausages, reduce heat to medium-low, and cover with a lid. Cook for 10 minutes.

3 While the sausages cook, prepare the slurry. In a medium bowl, whisk together the arrowroot flour and cold water until well combined.

4 Add the slurry to the pan and stir, scraping up any brown bits from the bottom. Increase heat and bring to a boil. Once boiling, remove from heat and cover.

5 Place the steamed cauliflower in a food processor and process until it reaches the consistency of mashed potatoes.

6 In a medium saucepan, melt butter over medium heat. Add garlic and Italian seasoning and cook for 1 minute, until fragrant. Add the cauliflower, nutmeg, salt, and pepper. Stir together and cook for 2 to 3 minutes.

7 To assemble the meals, add 1 cup mashed cauliflower to each of 4 containers. Top with 2 sausages and divide the gravy evenly among the containers.

A light almond-flour batter gives cod a crispy coating, and homemade fries are roasted with garlic and seasonings.

Fish and Chips
with Sautéed Spinach

PREP TIME 15 minutes   **COOK TIME** 30 minutes   **MAKES** 4 servings   **SERVING SIZE** 1 assembled meal

NUTRITION PER SERVING Protein 27g / Carbohydrates 30g / Fiber 8g / Sugars 2g / Fat 30g / Calories 498

2 russet potatoes, cut into fries, about 1⅓lb (600g) in total

3 tbsp olive oil

5 garlic cloves, minced

½ tsp salt

½ tsp freshly ground black pepper

½ cup arrowroot flour

4 pieces cod or other firm-fleshed white fish, about 5oz (150g) each

½ cup unflavored soda water

½ cup almond flour

2 tbsp coconut oil

10oz (280g) baby spinach

Lemon wedges, to serve

½ cup **Ketchup** (see p17), to serve

1 Preheat the oven to 450°F (230°C) and line a baking sheet with parchment paper or foil. In a large bowl, toss the potatoes with 2 tbsp olive oil, 3 minced garlic cloves, ¼ tsp salt, and ¼ tsp pepper until well coated. Spread on the prepared baking sheet and bake for 25 to 30 minutes.
➥ *Return to Prep Day Action Plan while potatoes bake.*

2 Place the arrowroot flour in a shallow bowl. Coat the fish in the arrowroot flour, covering each piece on all sides.

3 Make the batter by whisking together the soda water, almond flour, and remaining ¼ tsp salt and ¼ tsp pepper.

4 In a large non-stick pan, melt coconut oil over medium-high heat. Dip the flour-coated fish in the batter, fully coating each piece, then place in the hot pan and cook for 3 to 4 minutes on each side, or until flaky. Transfer cooked fish directly to meal prep containers.

5 In the same pan, heat remaining 1 tbsp olive oil over medium heat. Add remaining 2 minced garlic cloves and cook for 30 seconds, until fragrant. Add the spinach and cook until wilted.

6 To assemble the meals, divide the fries and spinach among the 4 containers with the fish and add a wedge of lemon to each. Serve each meal with 2 tbsp ketchup.

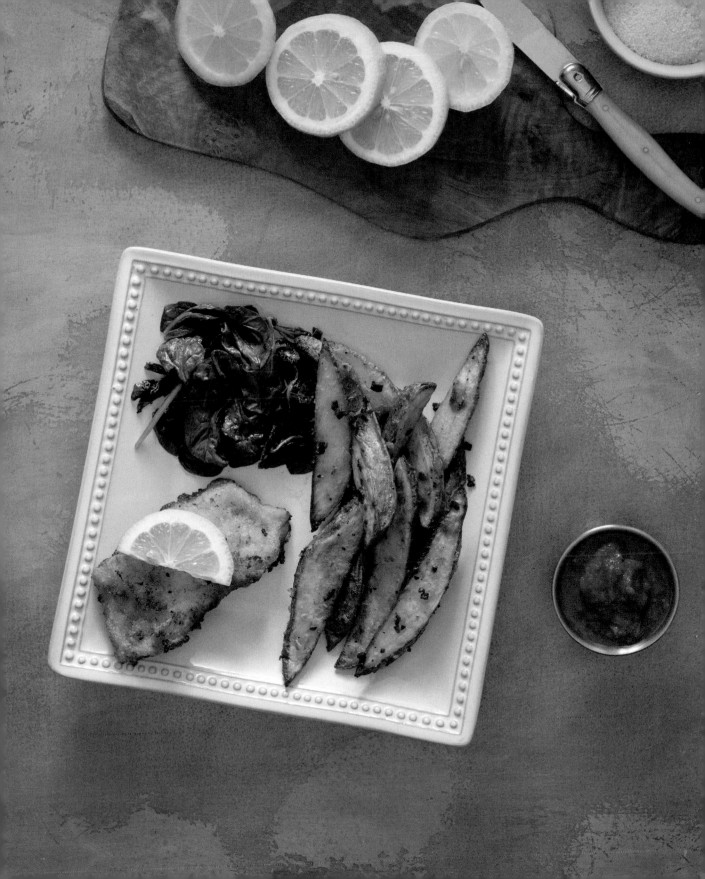

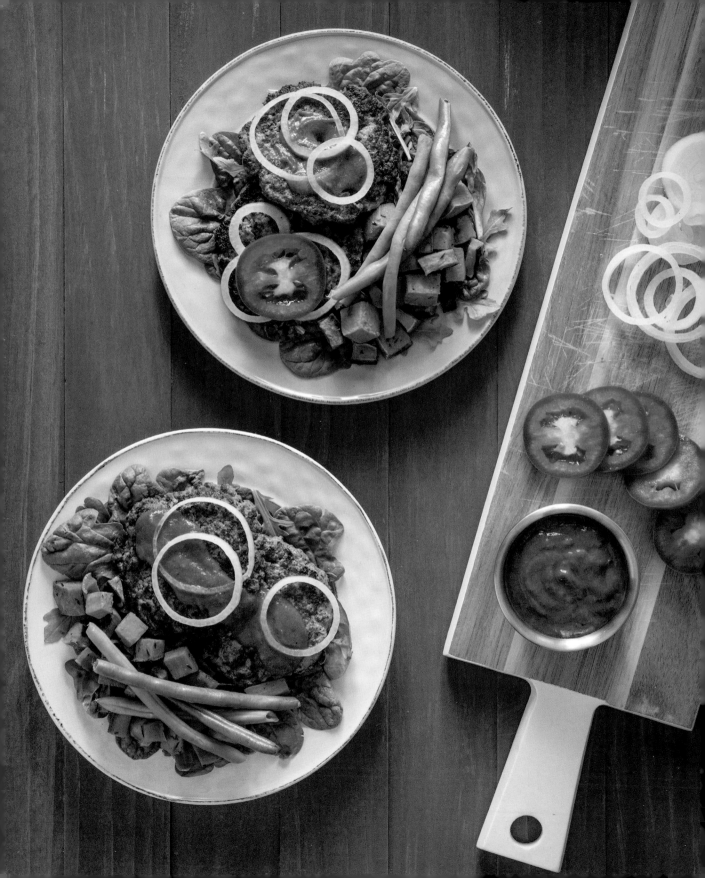

You don't need a bun for these juicy burgers, which are seasoned with mustard, garlic, and onion for exceptional flavor.

Beef Burgers
with Sweet Potatoes and Green Beans

PREP TIME 5 minutes   **COOK TIME** 30 minutes   **MAKES** 4 servings   **SERVING SIZE** 1 assembled meal

NUTRITION PER SERVING Protein 41g / Carbohydrates 27g / Fiber 6g / Sugars 4g / Fat 28g / Calories 524

2 sweet potatoes, diced, about 14oz (400g) in total

2 tbsp olive oil

1 tbsp chopped fresh thyme

½ tsp salt

½ tsp freshly ground black pepper

14oz (400g) fresh green beans, trimmed

1½lb (700g) 90% lean ground beef

2 large eggs

1 tbsp Dijon mustard

1 tbsp onion powder

1 tsp garlic powder

½ cup **BBQ sauce** (see p16)

TO SERVE (OPTIONAL)

Baby spinach or other greens

Sliced tomato

Sliced onion

1 Preheat the oven to 450°F (230°C) and line a baking sheet with parchment paper or foil. In a medium bowl, toss the sweet potatoes with 1 tbsp olive oil, thyme, ¼ tsp salt, and ¼ tsp pepper. Spread the potatoes on the prepared baking sheet and bake for 25 minutes.
➡ *Return to Prep Day Action Plan while potatoes bake.*

2 In a pot with a steamer insert, steam the green beans for 15 minutes, or until crisp-tender. Plunge the cooked beans into a bowl of ice water, then drain.
➡ *Return to Prep Day Action Plan while green beans steam.*

3 In the bowl used for the potatoes, mix together the ground beef, eggs, mustard, onion powder, garlic powder, and remaining ¼ tsp salt and ¼ tsp pepper. Using a ⅓-cup measure, scoop out the meat mixture and form into 8 patties.

4 In a large, non-stick pan, heat remaining 1 tbsp olive oil over medium-high heat. Add 4 patties to the pan and cook for 3 to 4 minutes until golden brown. Flip the patties, cover with a lid, and cook for another 4 minutes or until burgers reach desired level of doneness. Repeat for the second batch of 4 patties.

5 To assemble the meals, divide the green beans and sweet potatoes evenly among 4 containers. Add 2 burger patties to each container and top with 2 tbsp BBQ sauce and additional toppings, if using. (Note that nutrition per serving does not include greens, tomato, or onion.)

Homemade Takeout

With this week's meal prep, you get the taste and convenience of takeout without the expense and unhealthy ingredients. Instead of stopping for fried rice and beef with broccoli on the way home, it's already in your fridge, ready to enjoy.

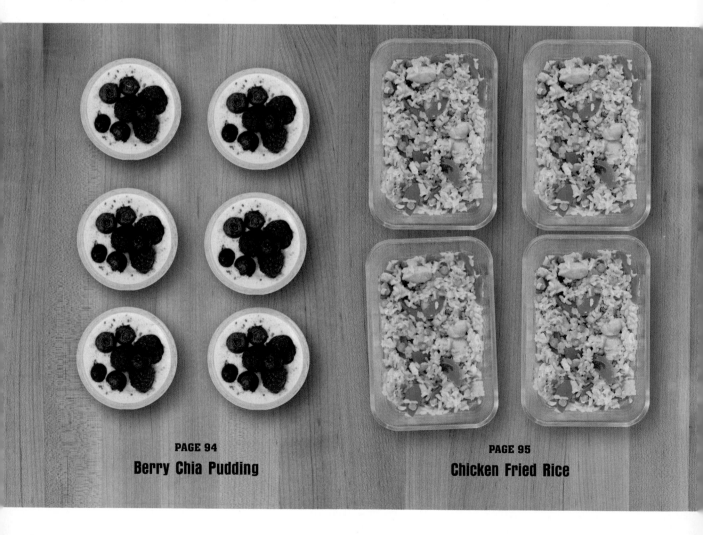

PAGE 94
Berry Chia Pudding

PAGE 95
Chicken Fried Rice

Coconut Aminos

Naturally gluten-free **coconut aminos** are a great substitute for soy sauce, with a savory-sweet flavor and 300 percent less sodium than most soy sauce brands.

Arrowroot Flour Slurry

A **slurry** is a combination of any vegetable starch and cold water. It can be mixed with pan juices to thicken gravies and sauces for cooked meats and stir fries.

SOMETHING TO MUNCH ON

- Cut extra carrot sticks and enjoy with almond butter throughout the week.

- Make your own fries by tossing potato wedges with olive oil, salt, and garlic and roasting at 450°F (230°C) for 25 minutes.

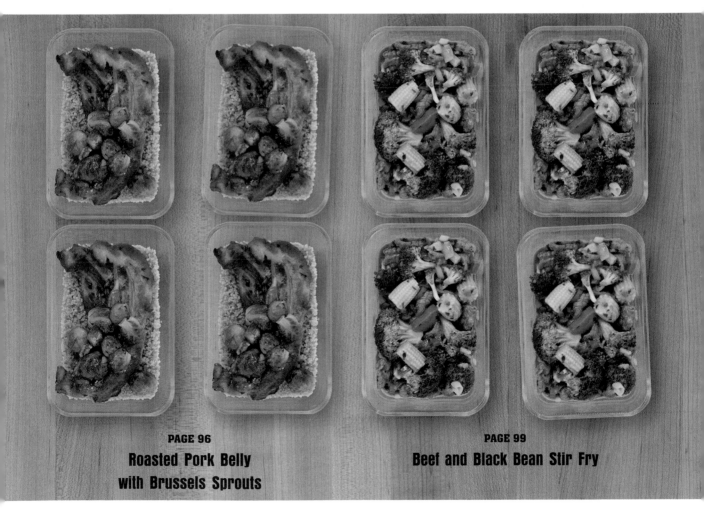

PAGE 96
**Roasted Pork Belly
with Brussels Sprouts**

PAGE 99
Beef and Black Bean Stir Fry

Prep Day Action Plan

EQUIPMENT

Chef's knife

Cutting board

Mixing bowls

Measuring cups

Measuring spoons

Large, non-stick sauté pan

Wok

Saucepan

Baking sheet

Aluminum foil or silicone baking sheet

Mesh sieve

Spatula

Food processor

Meal prep containers (12)

Small jars (6)

Food scale (optional)

 Homemade Takeout shopping list, p149

1 Preheat the oven to 400°F (200°C) and line a baking sheet with foil. Prepare basmati rice according to package directions. You'll need about ¾ cup uncooked rice to yield 2 cups cooked.

2 While the rice is cooking, slice 1¼lb (570g) pork belly into 8 pieces and prepare produce for the pork belly and stir fry.

For the pork belly:
2 garlic cloves, minced
1 tbsp minced fresh ginger
➡ Place in large bowl.

1lb (450g) Brussels sprouts, halved
➡ Place in medium bowl.

For the stir fry:
4 garlic cloves, minced
1 small yellow onion, diced
1 bunch scallions, diced, white parts only (set green parts aside)
➡ Place in medium bowl.

3 medium carrots, sliced into half-moons
1 head broccoli, cut into florets
11oz (300g) baby corn, halved
➡ Place in a medium bowl.

3 Check on the rice. When fully cooked, rinse in a sieve under cold water and spread on a baking sheet to cool.

Week at a Glance

 Day 1
Breakfast Berry Chia Pudding
Lunch Chicken Fried Rice
Dinner Roasted Pork Belly

 Day 2
Breakfast Berry Chia Pudding
Lunch Beef and Black Bean Stir Fry
Dinner Chicken Fried Rice

 Day 3
Breakfast Berry Chia Pudding
Lunch Roasted Pork Belly
Dinner Beef and Black Bean Stir Fry

4 Begin making the **pork belly (p96, steps 1–2).** Put the pork and Brussels sprouts in the oven and set a timer for 30 minutes.

5 Prepare the quinoa according to package directions. You'll need about ¾ cup uncooked quinoa to yield 2 cups cooked.

6 Make the black bean sauce for the **stir fry (p99, step 1).** Check the quinoa and remove from heat when cooked. When the timer goes off, complete the **pork belly (p96, steps 3–5).**

7 Slice 1lb (450g) top round roast into strips. Put the beef in a large bowl and prepare the **stir fry (p99, steps 2–6).**

8 Prepare ingredients for the fried rice.
1 small yellow onion, diced
4 scallions, diced, white parts only (set green parts aside)
➡ Place in small bowl.

1⅓lb (600g) skinless, boneless chicken breast, cubed
➡ Place in a medium bowl.

2 medium carrots, diced
¾ cup frozen green peas
➡ Place in a medium bowl.

9 Make the **chicken fried rice (p95, all steps)** and portion into containers. Then make the **chia puddings (p94, all steps).**

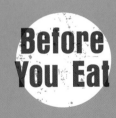

Before You Eat

Berry Chia Pudding
Serve well chilled and stir before eating.

Chicken Fried Rice
Heat if desired, or enjoy cold.

Roasted Pork Belly
Heat if desired, or enjoy cold.

Beef and Black Bean Stir Fry
Heat if desired, or enjoy cold.

Day 4
Breakfast Berry Chia Pudding
Lunch Chicken Fried Rice
Dinner Roasted Pork Belly

Day 5
Breakfast Berry Chia Pudding
Lunch Beef and Black Bean Stir Fry
Dinner Chicken Fried Rice

Day 6
Breakfast Berry Chia Pudding
Lunch Roasted Pork Belly
Dinner Beef and Black Bean Stir Fry

Chia seeds add subtle texture to this sweet, creamy pudding, which can be made with the seasonal berries of your choice.

Berry Chia Pudding

PREP TIME 5 minutes   **COOK TIME** 0 minutes   **MAKES** 6 jars   **SERVING SIZE** 1 jar

NUTRITION PER SERVING Protein 17g / Carbohydrates 22g / Fiber 12g / Sugars 10g / Fat 26g / Calories 390

2 13.5oz (400ml) cans coconut milk

¾ cup chia seeds

2 tbsp coconut sugar

6 tbsp undenatured whey protein

1 cup blueberries, plus extra to garnish

½ cup raspberries, plus extra to garnish

1 In a large bowl, stir together the coconut milk, chia seeds, coconut sugar, and whey protein until well combined. Fold in the blueberries and raspberries.

2 Divide the mixture evenly among 6 small jars or airtight containers, top with additional berries if desired, and refrigerate. Puddings will thicken as they chill, and are ready to eat after about 2 hours.

 What do chia seeds taste like?

Chia seeds don't have much flavor on their own, but they thicken the pudding and add texture. They're also a great source of antioxidants and omega-3 fatty acids.

Once you learn how quick and easy it is to make healthy chicken fried rice, you'll never need to order it again.

Chicken Fried Rice

PREP TIME 10 minutes   **COOK TIME** 15 minutes   **MAKES** 4 servings   **SERVING SIZE** 1 assembled meal

NUTRITION PER SERVING Protein 42g / Carbohydrates 32g / Fiber 3g / Sugars 5g / Fat 18g / Calories 467

4 tbsp olive oil

½ small yellow onion, diced

4 scallions, diced, white and green parts kept separate

2 large eggs

1⅓lb (600g) skinless, boneless chicken breast, cubed

½ tsp salt

¼ tsp freshly ground black pepper

4 tbsp coconut aminos (or liquid aminos or soy sauce)

2 medium carrots, diced

¾ cup frozen green peas

2 cups cooked brown basmati rice, cooled

1 In a large wok or non-stick sauté pan, heat 2 tbsp olive oil over medium-high heat. Add the onion and white parts of the scallions. Sauté for 2 minutes.

2 Push the onions to the side of the wok, and crack in the eggs. Using a spatula or wooden spoon, stir the eggs until scrambled and fully cooked. Mix with the onion.

3 Push the eggs and onion to the side, add the cubed chicken to the wok, and season with salt and pepper. Cook, stirring occasionally, until the chicken begins to turn white, about 3 minutes. Reduce heat to medium, add 2 tbsp coconut aminos, and stir. Cook for 4 minutes.

4 Add the carrots, peas, and the green parts of the scallions. Stir and cook for 2 minutes. Add the cooked basmati rice and stir. Add remaining 2 tbsp olive oil and remaining 2 tbsp coconut aminos. Stir and remove from heat.

5 To assemble the meals, divide the fried rice evenly among 4 meal prep containers.

Brussels sprouts are roasted with pork belly and finished with red wine vinegar for an irresistably tangy flavor.

Roasted Pork Belly
with Brussels Sprouts

PREP TIME 10 minutes   **COOK TIME** 30 minutes   **MAKES** 4 servings   **SERVING SIZE** 1 assembled meal

NUTRITION PER SERVING Protein 27g / Carbohydrates 35g / Fiber 7g / Sugars 6g / Fat 32g / Calories 536

2 garlic cloves, minced

1 tbsp minced fresh ginger

2 tbsp low-sodium soy sauce

2 tbsp coconut sugar

1¼lb (570g) pork belly, cut into 8 slices

1lb (450g) Brussels sprouts, halved

¼ cup red wine vinegar

¼ cup water

2 cups cooked quinoa

1 Preheat the oven to 400°F (200°C) and line a rimmed baking sheet with a silicone baking mat or foil. In a large bowl, mix together the garlic, ginger, soy sauce, and coconut sugar. Add the pork belly and Brussels sprouts and mix until well coated.

2 Arrange the pork and Brussels sprouts on the prepared baking sheet. Roast for 30 minutes until Brussels sprouts are beginning to brown. Pork belly should be brown at edge and firm to the touch.
➥ *Return to Prep Day Action plan while pork and Brussels sprouts roast.*

3 When the pork is fully cooked, remove from the oven. Place 2 pieces of pork in each of 4 meal prep containers.

4 While the pan is still hot, toss the red wine vinegar with the Brussels sprouts. Add the water, toss again, and return to the oven for 5 minutes.

5 To assemble the meals, add ½ cup cooked quinoa to each of 4 containers, along with the pork. Remove the Brussels sprouts from the oven, give them a stir, and divide them evenly among the containers. Pour the pan juices evenly over top.

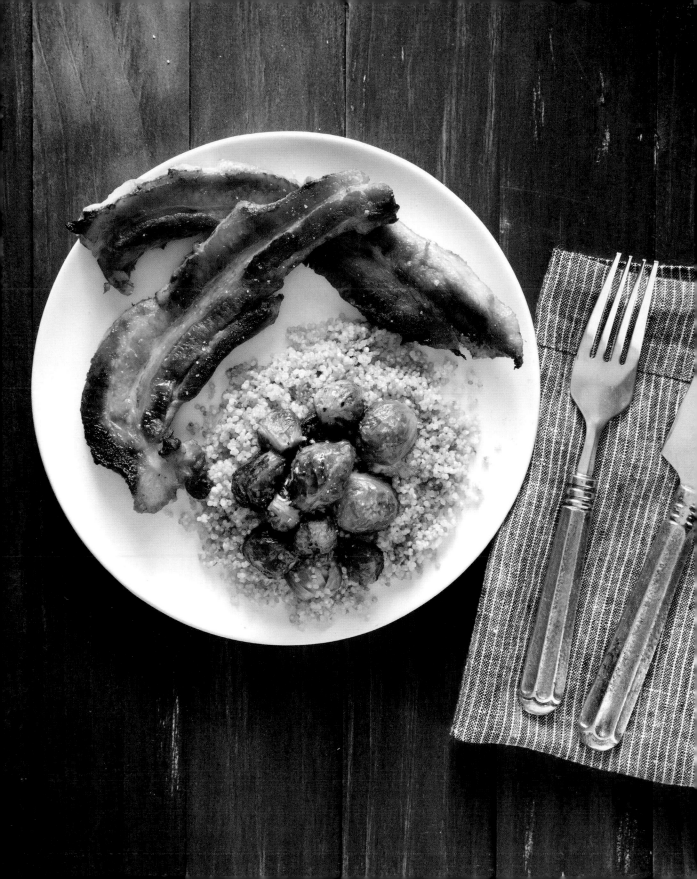

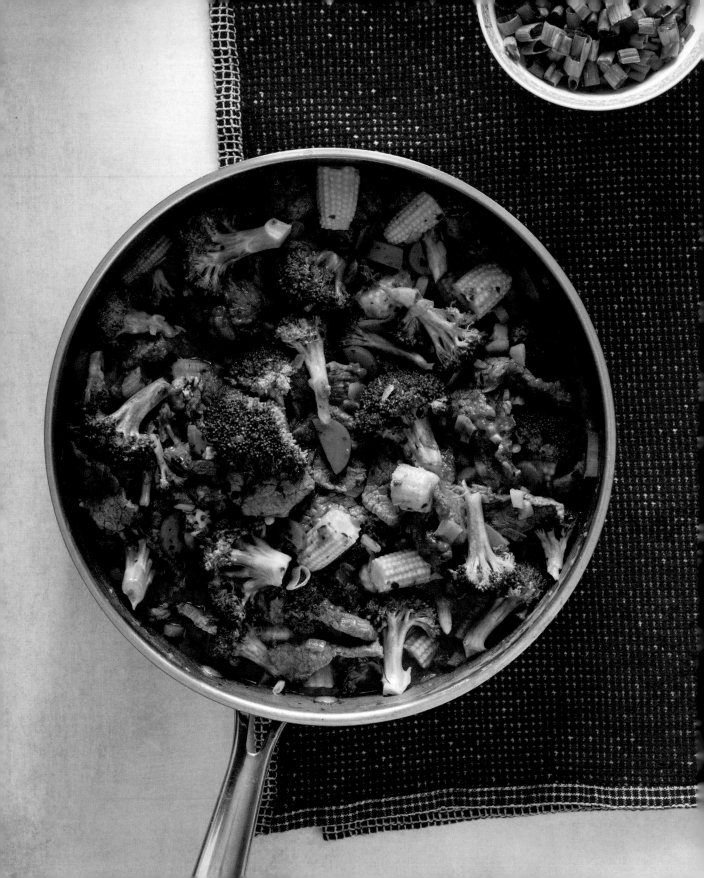

This version of beef and broccoli is flavored with a savory black bean sauce, and includes a colorful mix of vegetables.

Beef and Black Bean Stir Fry

PREP TIME 15 minutes   **COOK TIME** 15 minutes   **MAKES** 4 servings   **SERVING SIZE** 1 assembled meal

NUTRITION PER SERVING Protein 43g / Carbohydrates 40g / Fiber 10g / Sugars 10 / Fat 20g / Calories 512

FOR STIR FRY

1lb (450g) top round roast, sliced into thin strips

¼ cup + 1 tsp arrowroot flour

4 tbsp coconut oil

4 garlic cloves, minced

1 small yellow onion, diced

1 bunch scallions, chopped, white and green parts kept separate

3 medium carrots, sliced into half-moons

1 head broccoli, cut into florets

11oz (300g) baby corn, halved

½ cup cold water

2½ cups low-sodium beef stock

FOR BLACK BEAN PASTE

15oz (425g) can black beans, drained and rinsed

¼ cup coconut aminos (or liquid aminos or low-sodium soy sauce)

1 To make the black bean paste, blend black beans and coconut aminos in a food processor until a chunky paste forms. Transfer to an airtight container and refrigerate.
➡ *Return to Prep Day Action Plan.*

2 In a large bowl, toss the beef with ¼ cup arrowroot flour until the beef is well coated on all sides.

3 In a wok, melt 2 tbsp coconut oil over medium-high heat. Add the garlic, onion, and the white parts of scallions. Sauté for 2 to 3 minutes or until golden brown. Add the carrots, broccoli, and baby corn. Sauté for 2 to 3 minutes, then transfer the vegetables to a bowl and set aside.

4 Return the wok to the burner and melt remaining 2 tbsp coconut oil over medium heat. Add the beef and cook for 3 minutes, stirring to ensure that all sides cook evenly. Transfer the beef to the bowl with the vegetables.

5 To make the sauce, whisk the remaining 1 tsp arrowroot flour with cold water to make a slurry. Return the wok to the burner over medium-high heat, and add the slurry, beef stock, and ¼ cup black bean paste. Whisk until well combined and bring to a boil. Cook for 2 minutes before adding back in the beef and vegetables. Stir together until beef and vegetables are evenly coated with sauce, then remove from heat.

6 To assemble the meals, evenly divide the stir fry among 4 containers and garnish with the green parts of the scallion.

Asian Feast

From Thailand to India, this week's lunch and dinner meals draw inspiration from a variety of Asian culinary traditions. Indulge in creamy Butter Chicken and salty-sweet Shrimp and Tofu Pad Thai without the guilt or expense of eating out.

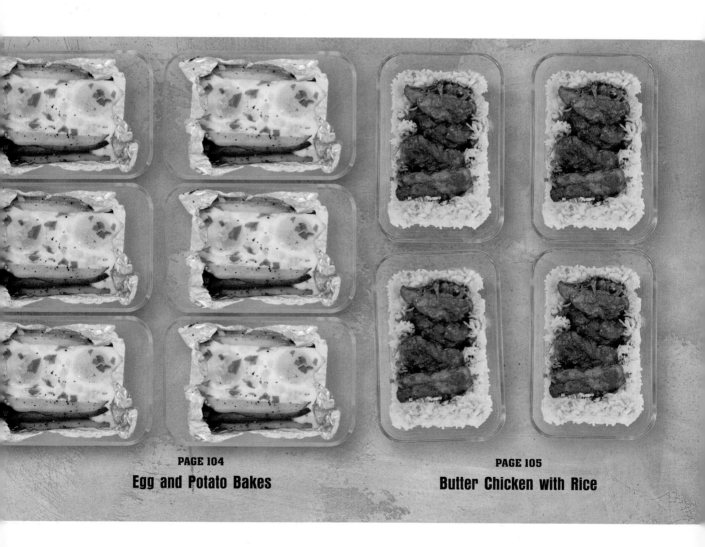

PAGE 104
Egg and Potato Bakes

PAGE 105
Butter Chicken with Rice

Foil Packets

Two meals this week are cooked in **foil packets**. This technique helps to ensure even cooking and prevents food from drying out. They also make portioning easy.

Protein Swap

If tofu isn't for you, replace the tofu in the **Shrimp and Tofu Pad Thai** with cubed **chicken breast**, or leave it out entirely.

SOMETHING TO MUNCH ON

- Top seaweed snack sheets with sliced avocado and a dash of hot sauce for a sushi-like snack.

- Edamame sprinkled with sea salt will satisfy snack cravings with fewer carbs and more protein than chips.

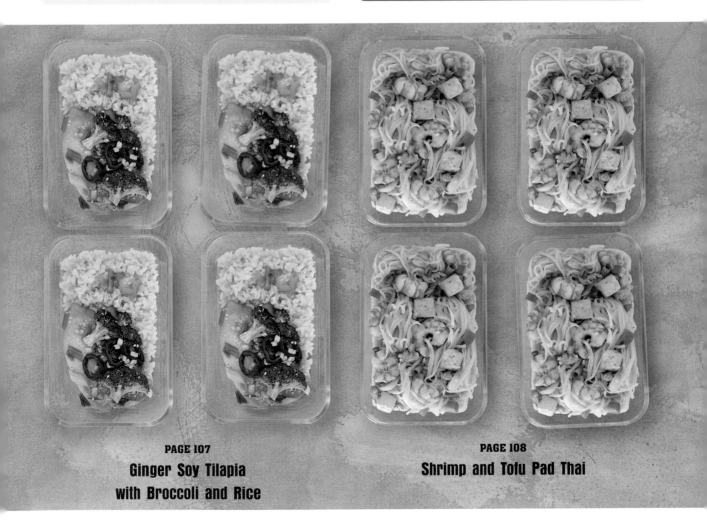

PAGE 107
Ginger Soy Tilapia with Broccoli and Rice

PAGE 108
Shrimp and Tofu Pad Thai

Prep Day Action Plan

EQUIPMENT
Chef's knife

Cutting board

Mixing bowls

Measuring cups

Measuring spoons

Large, non-stick sauté pan with lid

Wok

Saucepan

Spatula

Wooden spoon

Baking sheets (2)

Aluminum foil

Meal prep containers (18)

Food scale (optional)

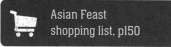

Asian Feast
shopping list, p150

1 Preheat the oven to 400°F (200°C). Cut 10 squares of aluminum foil, each about 12 x 12in (30 x 30cm). Wash and prepare the following ingredients.

For the egg and potato bakes:
3 russet potatoes, cut into thin wedges
➡ Place in a medium bowl.

For the chicken:
1 small yellow onion, diced
4 garlic cloves, minced
➡ Place in a small bowl.

1 tbsp ground cumin
1 tbsp chili powder
1 tbsp garam masala
1 tbsp turmeric
2 tsp ground ginger
¼ tsp salt
➡ Mix in a small bowl.

For the tilapia:
1 head broccoli, cut into florets
➡ Place in a medium bowl.

1 piece fresh ginger, peeled and minced
4 scallions, sliced
4 red chiles, sliced (optional)
➡ Place in a small bowl.

Week at a Glance

 Day 1

Breakfast Egg and Potato Bake

Lunch Ginger Soy Tilapia

Dinner Shrimp and Tofu Pad Thai

 Day 2

Breakfast Egg and Potato Bake

Lunch Butter Chicken

Dinner Ginger Soy Tilapia

 Day 3

Breakfast Egg and Potato Bake

Lunch Ginger Soy Tilapia

Dinner Shrimp and Tofu Pad Thai

2 Prepare the brown basmati rice according to package directions. You will need about 1¼ cups uncooked rice to yield 4 cups cooked rice.

3 While rice is cooking, begin preparing the **butter chicken (p105, steps 1–3).**

4 While the chicken simmers, prepare the foil packets for the **egg and potato bakes (p104, step 2).** Set a timer for 25 minutes.

5 Check on the rice. When fully cooked, remove from heat and set aside to cool. When chicken has simmered for 10 minutes, remove from heat and portion into containers along with the rice.

6 Prepare the foil packets for the **ginger soy tilapia (p107, steps 2–3).** Set a timer for 15 minutes. When you put the fish in the oven, check on the egg and potato bakes and remove if fully cooked.

7 Clear your workspace and prepare the ingredients for the pad thai. If necessary, defrost the shrimp in a sieve under cold running water. Mince 4 garlic cloves, slice 4 scallions, and cube 8oz (225g) extra-firm tofu. Make the **pad thai (p108, all steps).**

8 Remove the fish from the oven and transfer to meal prep containers.

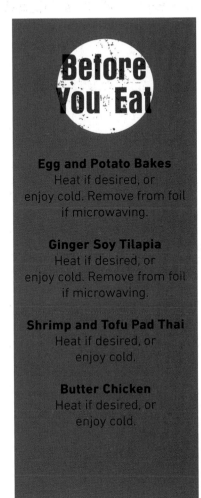

Before You Eat

Egg and Potato Bakes
Heat if desired, or enjoy cold. Remove from foil if microwaving.

Ginger Soy Tilapia
Heat if desired, or enjoy cold. Remove from foil if microwaving.

Shrimp and Tofu Pad Thai
Heat if desired, or enjoy cold.

Butter Chicken
Heat if desired, or enjoy cold.

Day 4
Breakfast Egg and Potato Bake
Lunch Butter Chicken
Dinner Ginger Soy Tilapia

Day 5
Breakfast Egg and Potato Bake
Lunch Shrimp and Tofu Pad Thai
Dinner Butter Chicken

Day 6
Breakfast Egg and Potato Bake
Lunch Butter Chicken
Dinner Shrimp and Tofu Pad Thai

This simple method results in tender, seasoned potato wedges topped with perfectly cooked eggs.

Egg and Potato Bakes

PREP TIME 10 minutes   **COOK TIME** 45 minutes   **MAKES** 6 packets   **SERVING SIZE** 1 packet

NUTRITION PER SERVING Protein 16g / Carbohydrates 29g / Fiber 3g / Sugars 0g / Fat 23g / Calories 390

3 russet potatoes, cut into thin wedges, about 1¾lb (800g) total

¼ cup + 2 tbsp olive oil

1 tbsp dried Italian seasoning

½ tsp salt

½ tsp freshly ground black pepper

12 large eggs

Chopped scallions, to garnish

1 Preheat the oven to 400°F (200°C). Cut a sheet of aluminum foil into 6 pieces, each about 12 x 12in (30 x 30cm).

2 In a medium bowl, toss the potato wedges with olive oil, Italian seasoning, salt, and pepper until well coated. Place an equal portion of potatoes onto each piece of foil.

3 Create a packet by folding the foil around the potatoes so they are fully enclosed, and fold over the edges to seal. Place the packets on a baking sheet and bake for 25 minutes.

4 Remove the tray from the oven, open the foil packets, and crack 2 eggs on top of the potatoes in each packet. Top each portion with chopped scallions, season with salt and pepper, and refold the packet. Bake for another 18 to 20 minutes, until the eggs look firm and are no longer runny.

5 Without unwrapping them, place each foil packet in a meal prep container and refrigerate.

Chicken becomes deliciously tender when simmered in a rich, creamy sauce with coconut milk and robust, warming spices.

Butter Chicken
with Rice

PREP TIME 10 minutes   **COOK TIME** 20 minutes   **MAKES** 4 servings   **SERVING SIZE** 1 assembled meal

NUTRITION PER SERVING Protein 30g / Carbohydrates 23g / Fiber 2g / Sugars 2g / Fat 45g / Calories 617

1 tbsp coconut oil

1 small yellow onion, diced

4 garlic cloves, minced

4 boneless, skinless chicken thighs, each trimmed and cut into 4 pieces

6 tbsp butter

14oz (414ml) can full-fat coconut milk

1 tbsp ground cumin

1 tbsp chili powder

1 tbsp garam masala

1 tbsp turmeric

2 tsp ground ginger

¼ tsp salt

2 cups cooked brown basmati rice

1 In a large wok, melt coconut oil over high heat. Add the onion and garlic and sauté for 3 minutes or until golden brown.

2 Add the chicken and cook until golden brown, about 3 minutes on each side. Transfer to a plate and set aside.

3 Add the butter to the hot pan. Once melted, stir in the coconut milk, cumin, chili powder, garam masala, turmeric, ginger, and salt. Bring to a boil, then reduce heat to low, add the chicken back in, and simmer for 10 minutes.

4 To assemble the meals, add ½ cup cooked rice to each of 4 meal prep containers, and divide the chicken mixture evenly among the containers.

 Do you really use 6 tbsp of butter? That seems like a lot. Yes—it is called butter chicken, after all! Butter is high in fat, but fat is not bad for you, especially when it is balanced with fewer refined carbs and more protein.

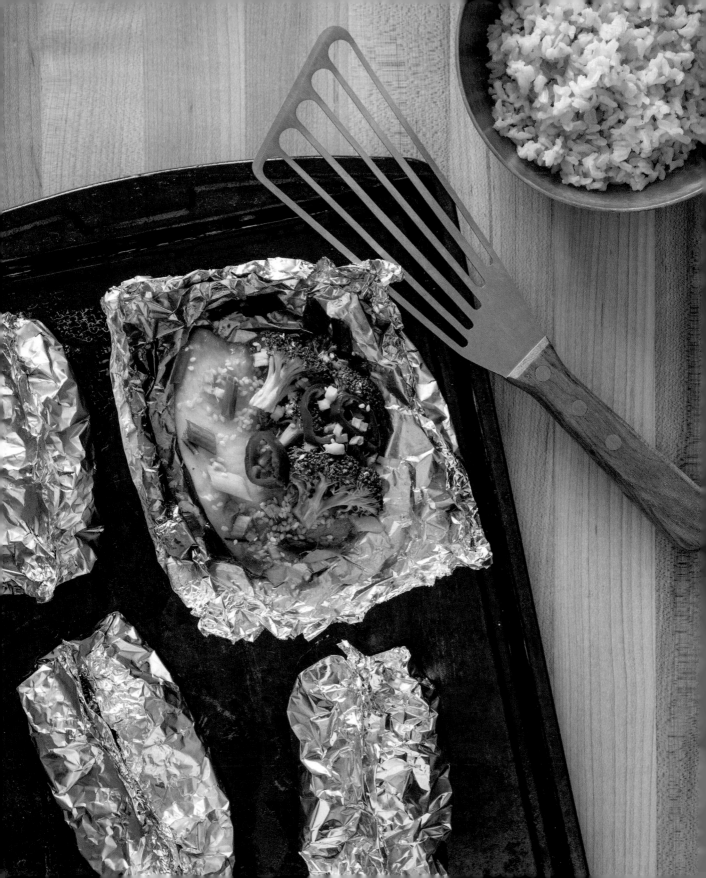

Making a foil packet allows the fish to gently steam, and seals in the flavors of ginger, soy sauce, and scallions.

Ginger Soy Tilapia
with Broccoli and Rice

PREP TIME 15 minutes   **COOK TIME** 30 minutes   **MAKES** 4 servings   **SERVING SIZE** 1 assembled meal

NUTRITION PER SERVING Protein 31g / Carbohydrates 34g / Fiber 3g / Sugars 2g / Fat 24g / Calories 476

4 pieces skinless tilapia, about 5oz (150g) each

1 head broccoli, cut into florets

4 tbsp low-sodium soy sauce

4 tbsp melted coconut oil

2 tbsp sesame seeds

1in (2.5cm) piece fresh ginger, peeled and minced

4 scallions, chopped

4 red chili peppers, such as cayenne, thinly sliced (optional)

2 cups cooked brown basmati rice

1 Preheat the oven to 400°F (200°C). Cut a sheet of aluminum foil into 4 pieces, each about 12 x 12in (30 x 30cm).

2 To assemble the packets, place 1 piece of fish in the center of each foil square. Arrange an equal portion of broccoli florets next to each piece of fish, and drizzle each serving with with 1 tbsp soy sauce and 1 tbsp coconut oil. Top each serving with sesame seeds, minced ginger, scallions, and sliced chilies (if using).

3 Create a packet by folding the foil around the fish and broccoli, crimping the edges to seal tightly. Place the packets on a baking sheet and bake for 15 minutes, until the fish is opaque and flakes easily with a fork.

4 To assemble the meals, place ½ cup cooked rice in each of 4 meal prep containers. To each container, add the fish and vegetables from one foil packet.

The original Thai noodle bowl is brimming with tofu and shrimp, and topped with chopped peanuts, cilantro, and lime.

Shrimp and Tofu Pad Thai

PREP TIME 5 minutes   **COOK TIME** 20 minutes   **MAKES** 4 servings   **SERVING SIZE** 1 assembled meal

NUTRITION PER SERVING Protein 34g / Carbohydrates 62g / Fiber 1g / Sugars 7g / Fat 27g / Calories 627

6 tbsp sesame oil

4 garlic cloves, minced

4 scallions, sliced, white and green parts kept separate

8oz (225g) extra firm tofu, cubed

2 large eggs

1lb (450g) raw shrimp, peeled and deveined

2 tbsp fish sauce

2 tbsp coconut sugar

2 tbsp low-sodium soy sauce

9oz (250g) Thai-style rice noodles

3 cups water

¼ tsp salt

TO SERVE (OPTIONAL)
Crushed peanuts

Chopped cilantro

Lime wedges

1 In a large, non-stick pan, heat sesame oil over medium-high heat. Add garlic and white parts of the scallions. Sauté for 2 minutes, then add cubed tofu and sauté for 2 minutes more.

2 Push all of the ingredients to the side of the pan and crack in the eggs. Using a spatula, stir the eggs until they are scrambled and fully cooked. Mix the eggs with the tofu and onion.

3 Add shrimp, fish sauce, coconut sugar, and soy sauce. Cook for 2 minutes, or until the shrimp is mostly pink.

4 Add noodles and water. Cover with a lid, increase heat to high, and cook for 3 minutes. When the noodles begin to soften, use a spatula to gently push them down into the liquid. Cook for 3 to 5 minutes more, stirring occasionally, until all of the liquid has been absorbed.

5 To assemble the meals, divide the pad thai evenly among 4 meal prep containers and garnish with green parts of scallions. Add crushed peanuts, chopped cilantro, and lime wedges to each meal, if using.

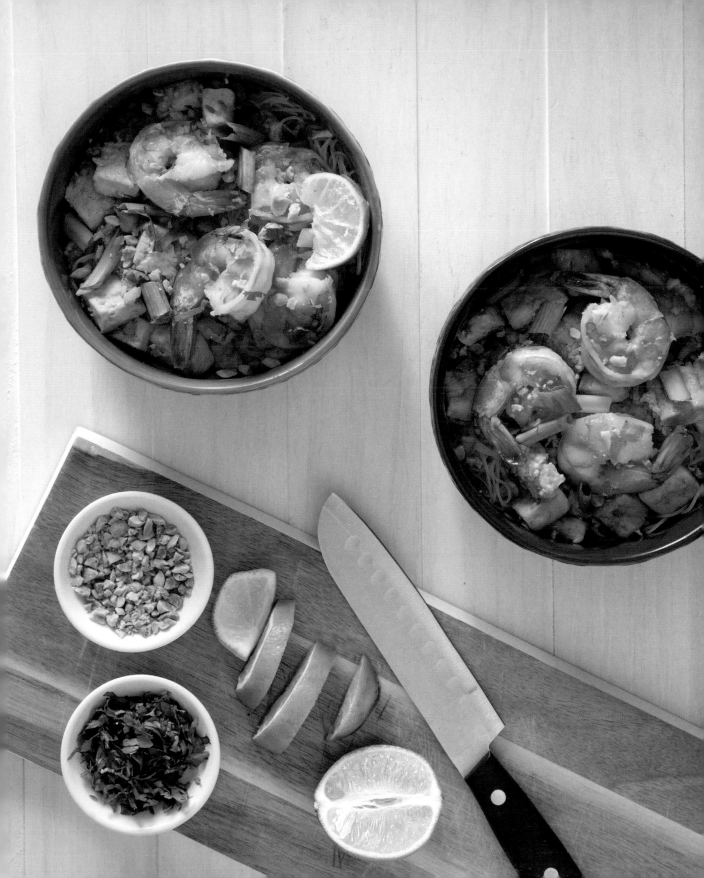

Bistro Classics

Come home to restaurant-quality meals at a fraction of the cost with this week's recipes for sirlion steak, spice-rubbed chicken, and pesto salmon. These impressive dishes will make even average weeknights feel like special occasions.

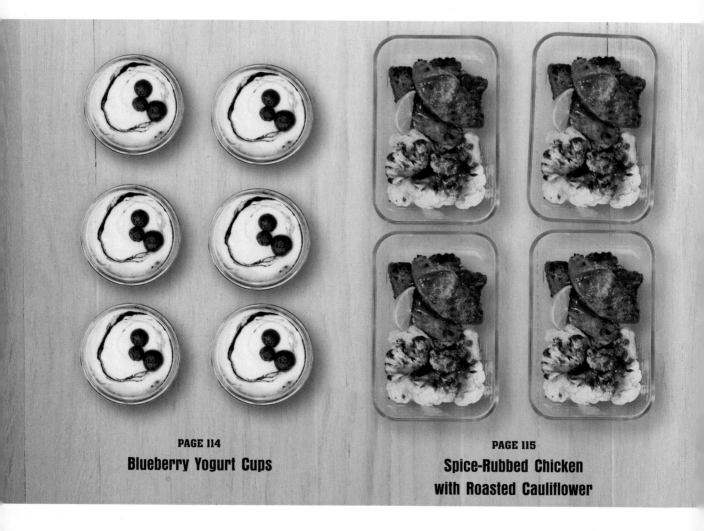

PAGE 114
Blueberry Yogurt Cups

PAGE 115
**Spice-Rubbed Chicken
with Roasted Cauliflower**

Broccolini

Also called "baby broccoli," **broccolini** is a cross between broccoli and the Chinese vegetable gai-lan. Broccolini has a narrow stalk and is milder and sweeter than regular broccoli.

Carb Swap

If you want to lower the carbs in the **Pesto Salmon** meal, replace the quinoa with **zucchini noodles** or **cauliflower rice**.

SOMETHING TO MUNCH ON

- Wrap sliced peaches or cataloupe with prosciutto for a sweet and salty snack.

- Roast extra cauliflower for snacking during the week.

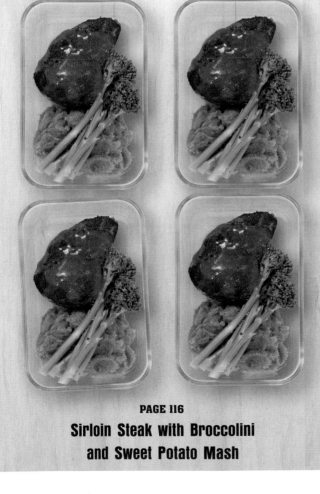

PAGE 116

Sirloin Steak with Broccolini and Sweet Potato Mash

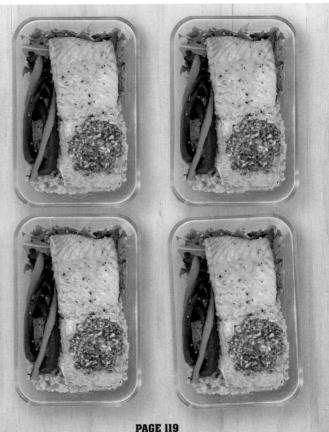

PAGE 119

Pesto Salmon with Peppers and Quinoa

Prep Day Action Plan

EQUIPMENT

Chef's knife

Cutting board

Mixing bowls

Measuring cups

Measuring spoons

Non-stick frying pan

Large pot

Pot with steamer insert

Saucepans (2)

Baking sheets (2)

Aluminum foil or parchment paper

Spatula

Whisk

Peeler

Meal prep containers (12)

Jars (6)

Food scale (optional)

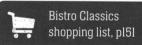

 Bistro Classics
shopping list, p151

1 Preheat the oven to 400°F (200°C). Line 2 baking sheets with foil or parchment paper. Prepare the following ingredients.

For the steak:
3 sweet potatoes, peeled and cubed
➡ Place in a large pot.

2 bunches broccolini, trimmed
➡ Place in a steamer insert.

For the salmon:
4 bell peppers, sliced
➡ Spread on a baking sheet.

For the chicken:
2 heads cauliflower, cut into florets
4 garlic cloves, crushed
➡ Spread on a baking sheet.

2 Slice 1⅓lb (600g) chicken breast and begin marinating for the **spice-rubbed chicken (p115, step 2).**

3 Prepare the cauliflower for the **spice-rubbed chicken (p115, step 1)** and the peppers for the **salmon (p119, step 1).** Put both trays in the oven and set a timer for 20 minutes.

4 In a small saucepan, begin cooking blueberries for the **yogurt cups (p114, step 1).**

Week at a Glance

Day 1
Breakfast Blueberry Yogurt Cup
Lunch Pesto Salmon
Dinner Sirloin Steak

Day 2
Breakfast Blueberry Yogurt Cup
Lunch Spice-Rubbed Chicken
Dinner Pesto Salmon

Day 3
Breakfast Blueberry Yogurt Cup
Lunch Sirloin Steak
Dinner Pesto Salmon

5 Prepare quinoa according to package directions. You will need about ¾ cup uncooked quinoa to yield 2 cups cooked.

6 While the blueberries and quinoa cook, cover the sweet potatoes with water and bring to a boil. Set up the steamer and begin steaming the broccolini. You will now have 4 pots on the stove.

7 When the blueberries begin to thicken, remove from heat. Assemble **yogurt cups (p114, steps 2–3)**.

8 When the timer goes off, cover the cooked quinoa and set aside. Remove the cauliflower from the oven and set aside to cool. Let the peppers cook for another 5 to 10 minutes.

9 When the broccolini is done, divide evenly among 4 meal prep containers. Mash the sweet potatoes for the **steak (p116, step 1)** and divide evenly among the containers with the broccolini.

10 Remove the peppers from the oven. Prepare the **salmon (p119, step 2)**. Set a timer for 10 minutes. Make the **quick pesto (p16, all steps)** and assemble the salmon meals.

11 Prepare the **steak (p116, steps 3–5)**. Add to the containers with the sweet potatoes and broccolini.

12 Prepare the **spice-rubbed chicken (p115, steps 3–6)**. Then assemble the **yogurt cups (p114, step 3)**.

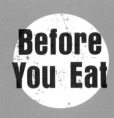

Before You Eat

Blueberry Yogurt Cups
Serve well chilled, and stir before eating.

Pesto Salmon
Heat if desired, or enjoy cold. If heating, remove arugula and pesto.

Sirloin Steak
Heat if desired, or enjoy cold. If heating, take care not to overcook steak.

Spice-Rubbed Chicken
Heat if desired, or enjoy cold.

Day 4
Breakfast Blueberry Yogurt Cup
Lunch Pesto Salmon
Dinner Spice-Rubbed Chicken

Day 5
Breakfast Blueberry Yogurt Cup
Lunch Sirloin Steak
Dinner Spice-Rubbed Chicken

Day 6
Breakfast Blueberry Yogurt Cup
Lunch Spice-Rubbed Chicken
Dinner Sirloin Steak

Any type of frozen berry can be used to create your own fruit-on-the-bottom yogurt with this simple technique.

Blueberry Yogurt Cups

PREP TIME 2 minutes　　**COOK TIME** 10 minutes　　**MAKES** 6 jars　　**SERVING SIZE** 1 jar

NUTRITION PER SERVING Protein 21g / Carbohydrates 20g / Fiber 3g / Sugars 15g / Fat 9g / Calories 245

3 cups frozen blueberries

½ cup water

6 cups plain, full-fat Greek yogurt

Fresh blueberries, to garnish (optional)

1 In a small saucepan, combine the frozen blueberries and water. Bring to a boil over medium-high heat, then reduce heat to low and cook for 5 to 6 minutes, stirring occasionally, until berries begin to break down and thicken.
➡ *Return to Prep Day Action Plan while blueberries cook.*

2 Divide the cooked blueberries evenly among 6 jars and let cool to room temperature. (To speed cooling, you can put the jars in the freezer, uncovered, for 5 minutes.)

3 Once the blueberries are cool, add 1 cup yogurt to each jar and top with fresh blueberries, if desired.

 Why is it important to use full-fat yogurt? Don't fear fat! Full-fat dairy products are more satiating than low-fat varieties, and keep you feeling full longer.

Cauliflower and garlic are irresistable when roasted and paired with chicken that has marinated in lime juice and spices.

Spice-Rubbed Chicken
with Roasted Cauliflower

PREP TIME 10 minutes   **COOK TIME** 20 minutes   **MAKES** 4 servings   **SERVING SIZE** 1 assembled meal

NUTRITION PER SERVING Protein 40g / Carbohydrates 14g / Fiber 6g / Sugars 6g / Fat 27g / Calories 459

2 heads cauliflower, cut into florets, about 2lb (1kg) in total

4 garlic cloves, minced

2 tbsp olive oil

1⅓lb (600g) skinless, boneless chicken breast, sliced

Juice of 1 lime

1 tsp ground cumin

1 tsp turmeric

1 tsp smoked paprika

2 tbsp coconut oil

1 tbsp arrowroot flour

½ cup cold water

4 tbsp butter

1 Preheat the oven to 400°F (200°C) and line a baking sheet with parchment paper or foil. Spread the cauliflower and garlic on the baking sheet and drizzle with olive oil, tossing to coat. Place in the oven and roast for 20 minutes.
➡ *Return to Prep Day Action Plan while cauliflower roasts.*

2 In a large bowl, toss the sliced chicken with the lime juice, cumin, turmeric, and paprika until well coated.
➡ *Return to Prep Day Action Plan while chicken marinates.*

3 In a large non-stick pan, melt the coconut oil over high heat. Add the chicken to the pan, spreading it out evenly, and cook for 3 to 4 minutes.

4 While the chicken cooks, combine the arrowroot powder and cold water in a small bowl and whisk to make a slurry.

5 Flip the chicken to the other side, pour in the slurry, and cover with a lid. Cook for 3 minutes, then remove the pan from the heat and add the butter. Stir until the butter has completely melted.

6 To assemble the meals, divide the chicken and cauliflower evenly among 4 containers, and pour sauce over top.

Juicy seared sirlion is topped with a tangy sauce and served with cumin-spiced sweet potato and fresh broccolini.

Sirloin Steak
with Broccolini and Sweet Potato Mash

PREP TIME 10 minutes   **COOK TIME** 30 minutes   **MAKES** 4 servings   **SERVING SIZE** 1 assembled meal

NUTRITION PER SERVING Protein 44g / Carbohydrates 37g / Fiber 7g / Sugars 8g / Fat 25g / Calories 549

3 medium sweet potatoes, peeled and cubed, about 1⅓lb (600g) in total

1 tbsp ground cumin

Salt and freshly ground black pepper

2 bunches broccolini

4 sirlion steaks, about 5oz (150g) each

1 tbsp coconut oil

1 tbsp arrowroot flour

½ cup cold water

1 tbsp tomato paste

1 tbsp apple cider vinegar

1 Place the sweet potatoes in a large pot and cover with water. Bring to a boil over high heat. Cook for 10 minutes or until easily pierced with a fork. Drain the water and return potatoes to the pot. Sprinkle with cumin, salt, and pepper, and mash until seasonings are incorporated.
➡ *Return to Prep Day Action Plan.*

2 In a pot with a steamer insert, steam the broccolini for 8 minutes, until bright green and crisp-tender.

3 Season steaks on both sides with salt and pepper. In a non-stick frying pan, melt the coconut oil over high heat. Add the steaks and cook for 3 to 4 minutes. Reduce heat to medium and cook for 3 to 4 minutes more. Flip the steaks, increase the heat to high, and cook for 3 to 4 minutes on the opposite side. Reduce heat to medium and cook for 3 to 4 minutes more. Remove pan from heat and let the steaks rest for 5 minutes, then transfer to a plate, leaving the juices in the pan.

4 In a small bowl, whisk together the arrowroot flour and cold water to make a slurry. In the same pan used for the steaks, stir the tomato paste and apple cider vinegar together with the pan juices, and bring to a boil over medium heat. Stir in the slurry, reduce the heat, and simmer for 3 minutes to form a sauce.

5 To assemble the meals, place 1 steak in each of 4 containers and divide the sweet potatoes, broccolini, and sauce evenly among the containers.

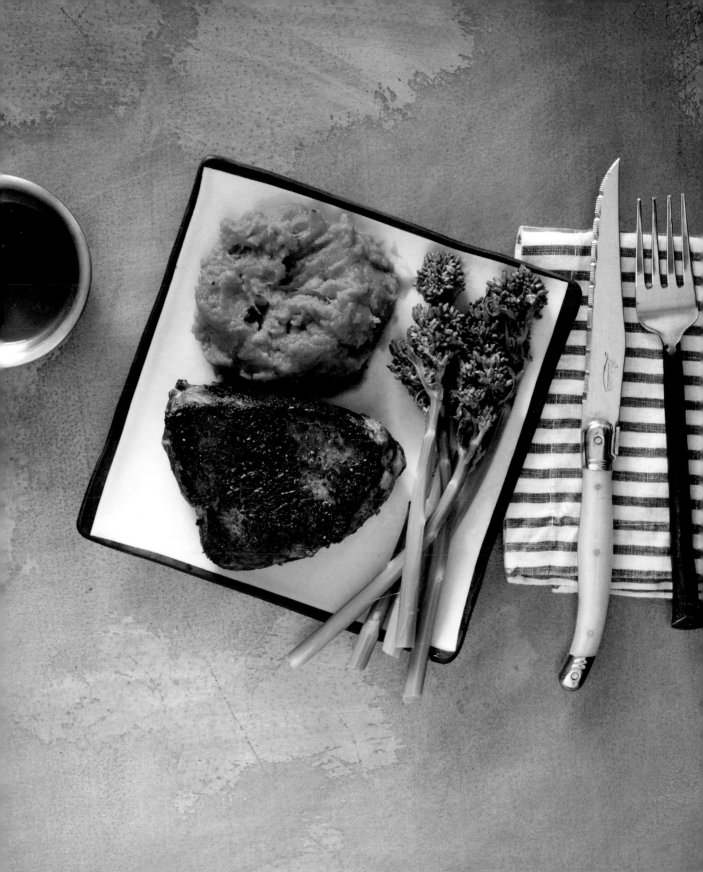

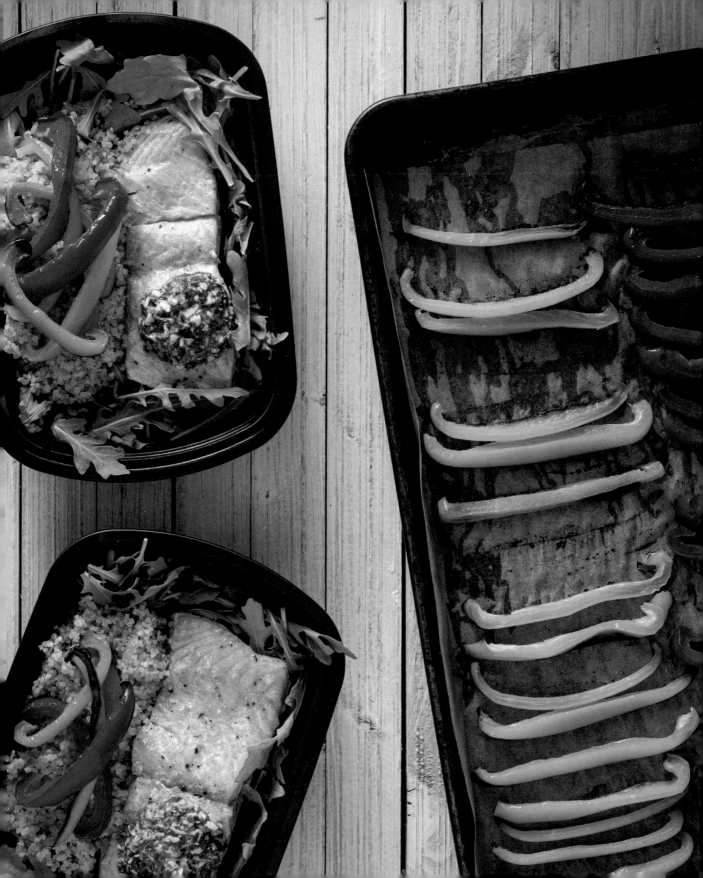

A squeeze of lemon juice and vibrant pesto add bright flavor to the roasted salmon and peppers in this colorful dish.

Pesto Salmon
with Roasted Peppers and Quinoa

PREP TIME 10 minutes   **COOK TIME** 40 minutes   **MAKES** 4 servings   **SERVING SIZE** 1 assembled meal

NUTRITION PER SERVING Protein 32 / Carbohydrates 29g / Fiber 7g / Sugars 8g / Fat 42g / Calories 622

4 pieces skinless salmon, about 4½oz (125g) each

4 bell peppers, any color, sliced

3 tbsp olive oil

Juice of ½ lemon

¼ tsp salt

¼ tsp freshly ground black pepper

2 cups cooked quinoa

2 cups baby arugula

½ cup **Quick Pesto** (see p16)

1 Preheat the oven to 400°F (200°C). Spread the bell peppers on a parchment-lined baking sheet and drizzle with 1 tbsp olive oil. Place in the oven and bake for 30 minutes.
➡ *Return to Prep Day Action Plan while peppers roast.*

2 Line a baking sheet with foil, folding up the edges to contain juices, and grease the foil with 1 tbsp olive oil. Arrange the fillets on the baking sheet and drizzle with remaining 1 tbsp olive oil. Squeeze lemon juice over top and season with salt and pepper. Bake for 10 minutes, or until salmon is firm to the touch.
➡ *Return to Prep Day Action Plan while salmon roasts.*

3 To assemble the meals, place ½ cup baby arugula and ½ cup cooked quinoa in each of 4 containers. Add a piece of salmon to each container, top with 2 tbsp pesto, and divide the roasted bell peppers evenly among the containers.

Viva Variety

This is the week for healthy, delicious recipes that break the mold with new cooking techniques and unexpected ingredients. Make polenta fries and zucchini fritters, try steamed bok choy, and bake turkey meatballs in a muffin pan.

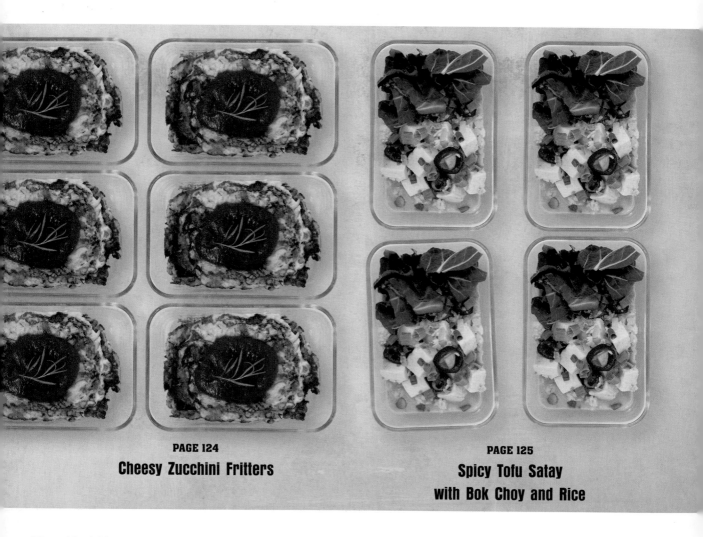

PAGE 124
Cheesy Zucchini Fritters

PAGE 125
**Spicy Tofu Satay
with Bok Choy and Rice**

Multi-Purpose Muffin Pan

Muffin pans aren't just for muffins! Cooking the **Turkey Meatballs** in the individual muffin cups keeps them moist and helps to prevent overcooking.

Vegetable Fritters

Almost any vegetable can be thinly sliced or grated and mixed with an egg batter to make a **fritter**, like this week's **Cheesy Zucchini Fritters**.

SOMETHING TO MUNCH ON

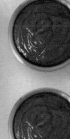

- Celery sticks with cream cheese and a sprinkle of pepper are an unexpectedly addictive snack.

- Make a quick egg salad by mixing chopped hardboiled eggs with mustard and serve in a lettuce wrap.

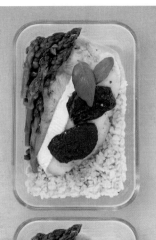
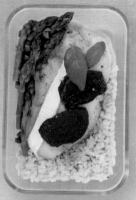
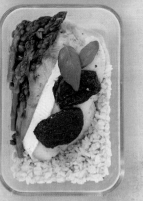
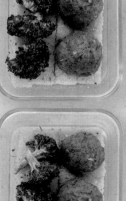
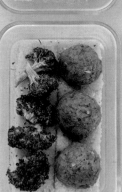
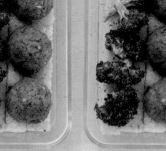
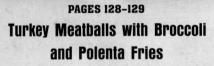

PAGE 127

Camembert Chicken with Asparagus

PAGES 128-129

Turkey Meatballs with Broccoli and Polenta Fries

Prep Day Action Plan

EQUIPMENT

Chef's knife

Cutting board

Mixing bowls

Measuring cups

Measuring spoons

Large wok

Non-stick frying pan

Pot with steamer insert

Medium saucepan

Baking sheets (2)

Aluminum foil

12-hole muffin pan

Grater

Whisk

Spatula

Food scale (optional)

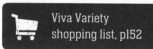

 Viva Variety
shopping list, p152

1 Prepare the rice for the Camembert chicken and tofu satay according to package directions. You will need about 1½ cups uncooked rice to yield 4 cups cooked.

2 While the rice is cooking, begin making the **polenta fries (p129, steps 1–3).** Place in the refrigerator for 30 minutes.

3 Prepare ingredients for the tofu satay.
13.5oz (385g) extra-firm tofu, cubed
➡ Place in a small bowl.

½ small yellow onion, diced
3 garlic cloves, minced
1in (2.5cm) piece fresh ginger, minced
1 red chili pepper, thinly sliced (optional)
➡ Place in a small bowl.

2 heads bok choy, trimmed
➡ Place in steamer insert.

4 Check the rice and remove from heat when cooked. Cover and set aside. Prepare the **tofu satay (p125, all steps).**

5 Preheat the oven to 400°F (200°C). While the oven heats, spread a dish towel over a large bowl and grate 4 zucchini squash into the towel. Squeeze out excess moisture. Dice 1 yellow onion and prepare the **zucchini fritters (p124, all steps).**

Week at a Glance

Day 1
Breakfast Cheesy Zucchini Fritters
Lunch Spicy Tofu Satay
Dinner Camembert Chicken

Day 2
Breakfast Cheesy Zucchini Fritters
Lunch Turkey Meatballs
Dinner Spicy Tofu Satay

Day 3
Breakfast Cheesy Zucchini Fritters
Lunch Camembert Chicken
Dinner Turkey Meatballs

6 Line a baking sheet with foil and finish the **polenta fries (p129, steps 4–5).** Put the fries on the top rack of the oven and set a timer for 30 minutes.

7 Once the polenta fries are in the oven, line a second baking sheet with foil. Cut 1 head broccoli into florets and prepare as directed for the **turkey meatballs (p128, step 2).** Put the broccoli on the lower rack and set a second timer for 20 minutes.

8 Cut the chicken breasts in half lengthwise, slice the Camembert cheese, and cut the asparagus into bite-size pieces. Prepare the **Camembert chicken (p127, steps 1–3).**

9 While the asparagus cooks, take the broccoli and polenta fries out of the oven. Divide them evenly among 4 meal prep containers. Finish the asparagus and assemble the Camembert chicken meals.

10 Prepare the **turkey meatballs (p128, steps 3–4)** and set a timer for 12 minutes. While the turkey meatballs bake, prepare the **BBQ sauce (p16, all steps).** When the turkey is done, add to the containers with the polenta fries and broccoli.

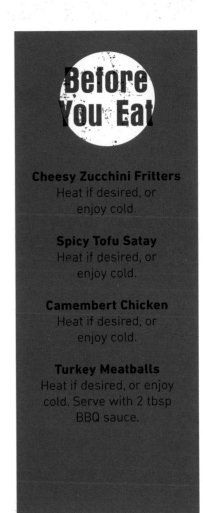

Before You Eat

Cheesy Zucchini Fritters
Heat if desired, or enjoy cold.

Spicy Tofu Satay
Heat if desired, or enjoy cold.

Camembert Chicken
Heat if desired, or enjoy cold.

Turkey Meatballs
Heat if desired, or enjoy cold. Serve with 2 tbsp BBQ sauce.

Day 4
Breakfast Cheesy Zucchini Fritters
Lunch Spicy Tofu Satay
Dinner Camembert Chicken

Day 5
Breakfast Cheesy Zucchini Fritters
Lunch Turkey Meatballs
Dinner Spicy Tofu Satay

Day 6
Breakfast Cheesy Zucchini Fritters
Lunch Camembert Chicken
Dinner Turkey Meatballs

Delicious hot or cold, these versatile fritters make a filling breakfast and are also great for snacking.

Cheesy Zucchini Fritters

PREP TIME 5 minutes　　**COOK TIME** 15 minutes　　**MAKES** 18 fritters　　**SERVING SIZE** 3 fritters

NUTRITION PER SERVING Protein 26g / Carbohydrates 13g / Fiber 8g / Sugars 9g / Fat 26g / Calories 420

4 medium zucchini squash, about 2lb (1kg) in total

10 large eggs

½ small yellow onion, diced

2 cups shredded mozzarella cheese, about 6oz (170g)

½ tsp salt

¼ tsp freshly ground black pepper

2 tbsp olive oil

½ cup marinara sauce, to serve

1 Spread a dish towel over a large bowl, and grate the zucchini over the towel. Use the towel to squeeze the liquid from the grated zucchini, getting it as dry as possible.

2 In a medium bowl, whisk eggs until the yolks and whites are well combined. Add the onion, zucchini, mozzarella, salt, and pepper. Stir until well combined.

3 In a large non-stick frying pan, heat ½ tbsp olive oil over high heat. Cook the fritters in batches, using a ⅓-cup measure to scoop the batter into the hot pan. Cook until the bottoms begin to brown, about 2 minutes, then use a spatula to carefully flip the fritters and cook for another 2 minutes. Repeat until the batter is gone, using ½ tbsp olive oil for each batch.

4 To assemble the meals, divide the fritters evenly among 6 meal prep containers. Top each meal with 2 tbsp marinara sauce.

Tofu is tossed in a spicy peanut sauce and served with hearty bok choy in this vegetarian twist on the Indonesian dish.

Spicy Tofu Satay
with Bok Choy and Rice

PREP TIME 5 minutes | **COOK TIME** 15 minutes | **MAKES** 4 servings | **SERVING SIZE** 1 assembled meal

NUTRITION PER SERVING Protein 22g / Carbohydrates 34g / Fiber 7g / Sugars 6g / Fat 40g / Calories 584

4 tbsp coconut oil

13.5oz (385g) extra firm tofu, cubed

3 garlic cloves, minced

½ small yellow onion, diced

1in (2.5cm) piece fresh ginger root, minced

1 red chili pepper, such as cayenne, thinly sliced (optional)

2 tbsp coconut aminos (or liquid aminos)

¼ cup all-natural peanut butter

13.5oz (400ml) coconut milk

1 cup water

2 heads bok choy, trimmed

2 cups cooked long-grain brown rice

2 scallions, sliced, to garnish

1 In a large wok, melt 2 tbsp coconut oil over high heat. Once the oil is hot, add the cubed tofu and fry until golden brown, about 5 minutes. Remove tofu from the wok and set aside.

2 In the same wok, heat remaining 2 tbsp coconut oil over high heat. Add the garlic, onion, ginger, and chili, if using. Sauté for 3 minutes.

3 Stir in the coconut aminos, peanut butter, coconut milk, and water, and bring to a boil. Once the mixture boils, reduce the heat to low and add the cooked tofu. Simmer for 3 minutes, and then remove from heat.

4 In a pot with a steamer insert, steam the bok choy for 4 minutes. Once bright green and crisp-tender, rinse under cold water for 1 minute to stop cooking.

5 To assemble the meals, place ½ cup cooked rice in each of 4 containers. Divide the tofu and bok choy evenly among the containers and top with sliced scallions.

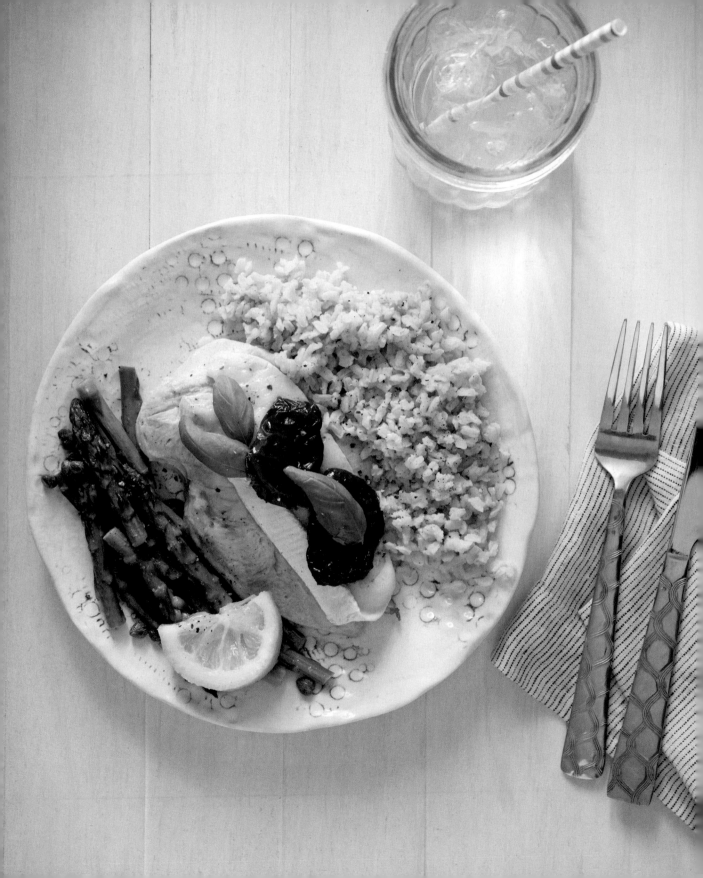

This elegant meal looks impressive, but couldn't be easier to make. Use Brie or mozzarella if you can't find Camembert.

Camembert Chicken
with Asparagus and Rice

PREP TIME 10 minutes   **COOK TIME** 20 minutes   **MAKES** 4 servings   **SERVING SIZE** 1 assembled meal

NUTRITION PER SERVING Protein 50g / Carbohydrates 28g / Fiber 3g / Sugars 3g / Fat 23g / Calories 519

2 tbsp coconut oil

2 skinless, boneless chicken breasts, about 1⅓lb (600g) total, halved lengthwise

8oz (225g) Camembert cheese

8 oil-packed sundried tomatoes, about 2oz (50g) in total

Handful of fresh basil leaves

1 bunch asparagus, about 7oz (200g), cut into bite-size pieces

2 tbsp capers

Juice of 1 lemon

2 cups cooked long-grain brown rice

1 In a large non-stick sauté pan, heat 1 tbsp coconut oil over high heat. Add the chicken, season with salt and pepper, and cook for 3 minutes. When the edges begin to turn white, flip over.

2 Reduce the heat to medium and top each piece of chicken with 2oz (56g) Camembert, 4 sundried tomatoes, and a few basil leaves. Cover the pan with a lid and cook for 3 minutes or until chicken is cooked through. Transfer the cooked chicken to 4 meal prep containers.

3 In the same pan, melt remaining 1 tbsp coconut oil over medium-high heat. Add the asparagus and capers, stir, and then cover with a lid. Cook for 10 minutes, stirring occasionally. Add the lemon juice, stir again, and remove from heat.
➡ *Return to Prep Day Action Plan while the asparagus cooks.*

4 To assemble the meals, add ½ cup cooked brown rice to each container with the chicken. Divide the asparagus evenly among the containers.

Garlic, oregano, and Dijon mustard flavor these tasty meatballs. Tender polenta fries and roasted broccoli complete the meal.

Turkey Meatballs
with Broccoli and Polenta Fries

PREP TIME 10 minutes　　**COOK TIME** 20 minutes　　**MAKES** 4 servings　　**SERVING SIZE** 1 assembled meal

NUTRITION PER SERVING Protein 34g / Carbohydrates 31g / Fiber 3g / Sugars 1g / Fat 25g / Calories 485

Coconut oil, for greasing pan

1 head broccoli, cut into florets, about 1lb (500g) total

1 tbsp olive oil

1 tbsp coconut aminos (or liquid aminos)

1⅓lb (600g) ground turkey

4 garlic cloves, minced

1 tbsp Dijon mustard

¼ tsp salt

¼ tsp freshly ground black pepper

1 tsp dried oregano

32 **Polenta Fries** (see p129)

¼ cup **BBQ Sauce** (see p16), to serve

1 Preheat the oven to 400°F (200°C) and line a baking sheet with parchment paper or foil. Grease a 12-hole muffin pan with coconut oil.

2 On the prepared baking sheet, use your hands to toss the broccoli florets with olive oil and coconut aminos. Spread out evenly and bake for 20 minutes.

3 In a medium bowl, mix together the ground turkey, garlic, Dijon mustard, salt, pepper, and oregano until well combined.

4 Scoop out about 2 tbsp of the ground turkey mixture and form into a ball with your hands. Place in the prepared muffin pan. Repeat to fill all 12 holes of the muffin pan. Bake for 12 to 15 minutes, until the turkey meatballs are firm to the touch.

5 To assemble the meals, place 8 polenta fries in each of 4 containers. Add 3 turkey meatballs to each container, and divide the roasted broccoli evenly among the containers. Serve with 2 tbsp BBQ Sauce.

A tasty alternative to potato fries, polenta fries made from seasoned cornmeal are easy to prepare and gluten free.

Polenta Fries

PREP TIME 30 minutes   **COOK TIME** 35 minutes   **MAKES** 32 fries   **SERVING SIZE** 8 fries

NUTRITION PER SERVING Protein 2g / Carbohydrates 23g / Fiber 2g / Sugars 0g / Fat 4g / Calories 136

1 tbsp coconut oil

1 cup polenta

4 cups water

½ tbsp dried rosemary

½ tbsp dried oregano

1 tsp salt

1 Line an 11 x 11in (28 x 28cm) pan with parchment paper and grease with 1 tbsp coconut oil.

2 In a medium pot, bring 4 cups water to a boil over high heat. Once boiling, slowly whisk in the polenta. Reduce the heat to low and continue to stir as it thickens, about 1 to 2 minutes. Remove from heat and stir in rosemary, oregano, and salt. The polenta should be thick but not too stiff to pour.

3 Using a spatula, spread the polenta into the pan. Dip the spatula in warm water to help spread the polenta evenly. Place in the refrigerator to cool for 30 minutes.
➡ *Return to Prep Day Action Plan while polenta cools.*

4 Preheat the oven to 400°F (200°C). When polenta has cooled, and feels firm to the touch, turn it out onto a cutting board. Cut the slab of polenta into 32 fries.

5 Line a baking sheet with foil and grease with coconut oil. Spread the polenta fries evenly on the baking sheet, and bake for 30 minutes, or until golden.

Meatless Meals

Vegetables are the star of this week's meals, which feature comfort foods without the meat. Even if you eat meat, taking a break from it occasionally can be good for your digestive system, and these hearty meals will keep you full and satisfied.

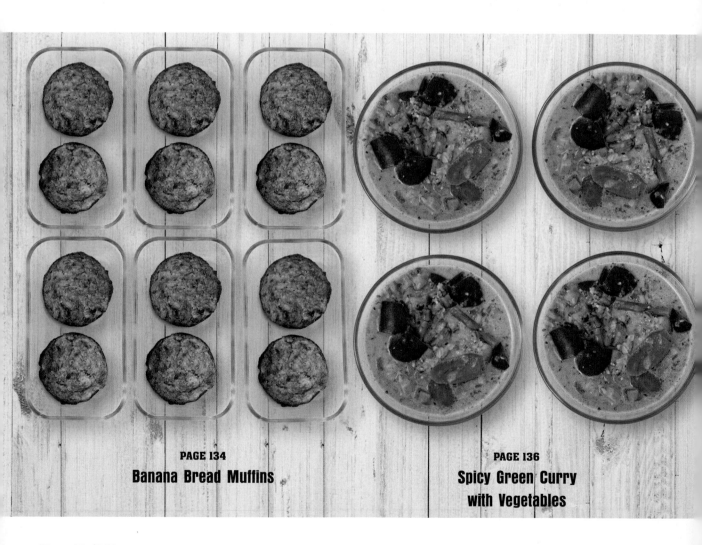

PAGE 134
Banana Bread Muffins

PAGE 136
Spicy Green Curry with Vegetables

Coconut Milk

Canned **coconut milk** is naturally lactose free, and gives curries a creamy consistency and slighty sweet flavor. Use the full-fat version for the best flavor and texture.

Flour Swap

If you are allergic to nuts, use **coconut flour** in place of **almond flour** for the **Banana Bread Muffins**.

SOMETHING TO MUNCH ON

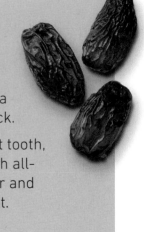

- Mashed avocado on whole-grain toast is a quick and filling snack.

- To satisfy your sweet tooth, stuff pitted dates with all-natural peanut butter and sprinkle with sea salt.

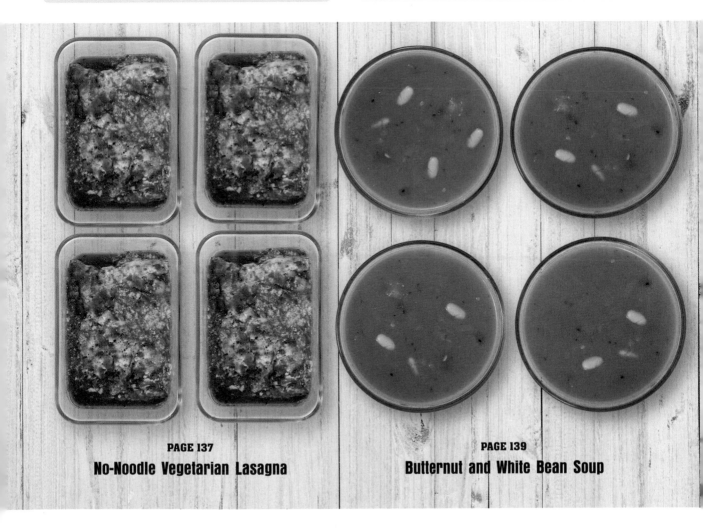

PAGE 137
No-Noodle Vegetarian Lasagna

PAGE 139
Butternut and White Bean Soup

Prep Day Action Plan

EQUIPMENT
Chef's knife

Cutting board

Mixing bowls

Measuring cups

Measuring spoons

Large wok with lid

9 x 9in (23 x 23cm) baking dish

12-hole muffin pan

Spatula

Aluminum foil

Food processor

Food scale (optional)

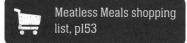 Meatless Meals shopping list, p153

1 Preheat the oven to 400°F (200°C). Wash and prepare ingredients for the lasagna:

1 eggplant, thinly sliced lengthwise into planks
8oz (225g) mushrooms, sliced
2 medium zucchini squash, thinly sliced lengthwise into planks

2 Assemble the **lasagna (p137, steps 1–4).** Place in the oven and set a timer for 30 minutes. While the lasagna bakes, clear your workspace and wash and prepare the ingredients for the curry and butternut soup.

For the soup:
4 garlic cloves, minced
1 small yellow onion, diced
4 sprigs fresh rosemary, chopped
➡ Place in a small bowl.

½ small butternut squash, diced
1 small sweet potato, diced
➡ Place in a medium bowl.

For the curry:
4–5 green chili peppers, stems removed and halved
1 shallot, quartered
4 garlic cloves, crushed
1in (2.5cm) piece fresh ginger root, peeled and roughly chopped
1 bunch cilantro, leaves and stems, roughly chopped
➡ Place in bowl of food processor.

Week at a Glance

Day 1

Breakfast Banana Bread Muffins

Lunch Butternut and White Bean Soup

Dinner No-Noodle Vegetable Lasagna

Day 2
Breakfast Banana Bread Muffins

Lunch Spicy Green Curry

Dinner Butternut and White Bean Soup

Day 3
Breakfast Banana Bread Muffins

Lunch No-Noodle Vegetable Lasagna

Dinner Spicy Green Curry

2 medium carrots, sliced
1 bell pepper red, diced
1 bunch asparagus, cut into bite-size pieces
1 eggplant, diced
➡ Place in a large bowl.

3 Make the curry paste and begin cooking the **curry (p136, steps 1–3).** When the timer goes off, stir the curry. Then remove the foil from the lasagna and return the pan to the oven. Set the timer for 15 minutes.

4 Begin cooking the **butternut and white bean soup (p139, steps 1–2).** While the soup simmers, check the curry. When the rice is fully cooked, portion into meal prep containers.

5 When the timer goes off, broil the lasagna for 2 minutes. Then remove from the oven and set aside to cool.

6 To finish the soup, carefully transfer the liquid to a blender and purée. Divide the beans evenly among 4 meal prep containers and ladle the soup over top.

7 Grease a 12-hole muffin pan with coconut oil and prepare the **banana bread muffins (p134, steps 1–4).**

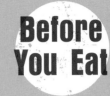

Before You Eat

Banana Bread Muffins
Best enjoyed at room temperature.

Butternut and White Bean Soup
Heat before serving. Top with ¼ cup ricotta and 2 tbsp pumpkin seeds.

Spicy Green Curry
Heat before serving, or enjoy cold.

No-Noodle Vegetable Lasagna
Heat before serving, or enjoy cold.

Day 4
Breakfast Banana Bread Muffins
Lunch Butternut and White Bean Soup
Dinner No-Noodle Vegetable Lasagna

Day 5
Breakfast Banana Bread Muffins
Lunch Spicy Green Curry
Dinner Butternut and White Bean Soup

Day 6
Breakfast Banana Bread Muffins
Lunch No-Noodle Vegetable Lasagna
Dinner Spicy Green Curry

These gluten-free muffins are so moist and tender, you'd never guess that they're also free of eggs, dairy, and added sugar.

Banana Bread Muffins

PREP TIME 5 minutes   **COOK TIME** 20 minutes   **MAKES** 12 servings   **SERVING SIZE** 2 muffins

NUTRITION PER SERVING Protein 6g / Carbohydrates 32g / Fiber 5g / Sugars 8g / Fat 19g / Calories 323

¼ cup melted coconut oil, plus extra for greasing

3 ripe bananas, about 13oz (375g) in total

¼ tsp salt

½ tsp baking powder

1 tsp baking soda

½ cup arrowroot flour

1 cup almond flour

½ cup old fashioned (rolled) oats

1 Preheat the oven to 400°F (200°C) and grease a 12-hole muffin pan with coconut oil.

2 In a large bowl, mash the bananas with a fork (some lumps are fine). Stir in the melted coconut oil.

3 Add the salt, baking powder, baking soda, arrowroot flour, almond flour, and oats. Mix until well combined.

4 Distribute the batter evenly among the holes of the prepared muffin pan. Bake for 18 to 20 minutes until the tops are brown. Allow the muffins to cool completely in the tin, then place 2 muffins in each meal prep container.

Can I make a loaf of banana bread instead of muffins?

Yes! To make a banana bread loaf, double the ingredients and bake in a greased 9 x 5in (23 x 12.5cm) loaf pan at 375°F (191°C) for 40 minutes.

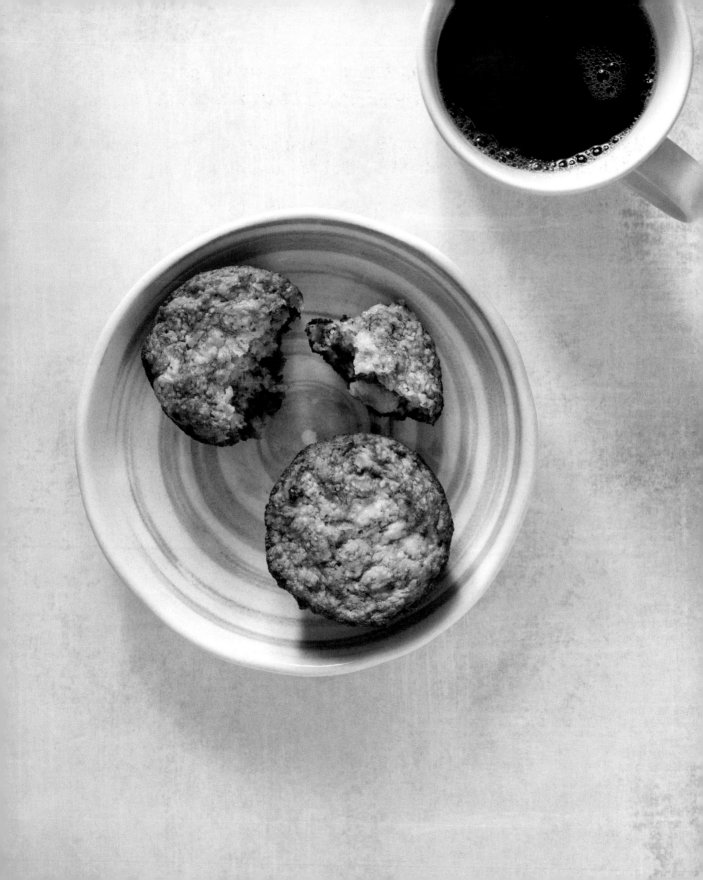

This simple one-pot dish gets its mild heat from a curry paste made with fresh jalapeños, garlic, ginger, and cilantro.

Spicy Green Curry
with Vegetables

PREP TIME 15 minutes **COOK TIME** 45 minutes **MAKES** 4 servings **SERVING SIZE** 1 assembled meal

NUTRITION PER SERVING Protein 12g / Carbohydrates 60g / Fiber 9g / Sugars 21g / Fat 40g / Calories 648

4–5 green chili peppers, such as jalapeños, stems removed and halved

1 shallot, quartered

4 garlic cloves, crushed

1in (2.5cm) piece fresh ginger root, peeled and roughly chopped

1 bunch cilantro, leaves and stems, roughly chopped

1 tbsp freshly ground black pepper

1 tbsp ground cumin

1 tbsp fish sauce

1 tbsp coconut oil

2 14oz (414ml) cans full-fat coconut milk

2 cups water

2 tbsp coconut sugar

2 medium carrots, sliced, about 7oz (200g) in total

1 red bell pepper, diced, about 7oz (200g) in total

1 bunch asparagus, cut into bite-size pieces, about 10½oz (300g) in total

1 eggplant, diced, about 14oz (400g) in total

1 cup uncooked brown rice

1 In a food processor, blend the chilies, shallot, garlic, ginger, cilantro, pepper, cumin, and fish sauce until ingredients are coarsely chopped and a rough paste forms.

2 In a large wok, heat the coconut oil over medium-high heat. Stir in the curry mixture and cook for 2 minutes. Whisk in the coconut milk, water, and coconut sugar, then add the carrots, pepper, asparagus, eggplant, and rice. Stir together.

3 Cover with a lid and cook for 45 minutes, stirring every 15 minutes. If the mixture becomes dry before the rice is cooked, add more water, ¼ cup at a time.
➡ *Return to Prep Day Action Plan while curry simmers.*

4 When the rice is fully cooked, divide the curry evenly among 4 meal prep containers.

TIP
For extra protein, add tofu or cooked, shredded chicken to the curry in step 2.

Sliced zucchini and eggplant stand in for noodles in this hearty layered casserole made with mushrooms and white beans.

No-Noodle Vegetable Lasagna

PREP TIME 15 minutes   **COOK TIME** 45 minutes   **MAKES** 4 servings   **SERVING SIZE** ¼ of pan

NUTRITION PER SERVING Protein 32g / Carbohydrates 43g / Fiber 15g / Sugars 5g / Fat 29g / Calories 561

1 eggplant, thinly sliced lengthwise into planks

4 garlic cloves, minced

14.5oz (425g) can cannellini beans, drained and rinsed

8oz (225g) mushrooms, sliced

2 cups marinara sauce

Handful of fresh basil leaves, roughly torn

2½ cups shredded full-fat mozzarella cheese

1 egg

1½ cups whole-milk ricotta cheese

Salt and freshly ground black pepper

2 medium zucchini squash (600g total), thinly sliced lengthwise into planks

1 Preheat the oven to 400°F (200°C). Line a 9 x 9in (23 x 23cm) baking dish with the sliced eggplant, covering the bottom as evenly as possible. Sprinkle with half of the minced garlic.

2 Spread the cannellini beans over the eggplant, then layer the mushrooms over the beans. Spread 1 cup marinara sauce evenly over the mushrooms, and top with half of the basil leaves and 1 cup mozzarella.

3 In a small bowl, mix together the egg and ricotta cheese. Season with salt and pepper, and spread the ricotta mixture evenly over the mozzarella. Layer the sliced zucchini over the ricotta and sprinkle with remaining garlic. Spread the remaining 1 cup marinara over the zucchini, and distribute the remaining basil and 1½ cups mozzarella over top. Season with freshly ground black pepper.

4 Cover with foil and place in the oven. After 30 minutes, remove the foil. Return to the oven for 15 minutes. To finish, broil the lasagna for 2 minutes or until the cheese is browned.

5 Refrigerate lasagna for 1 hour to cool completely before cutting into 4 pieces. Place 1 piece into each of 4 meal prep containers.

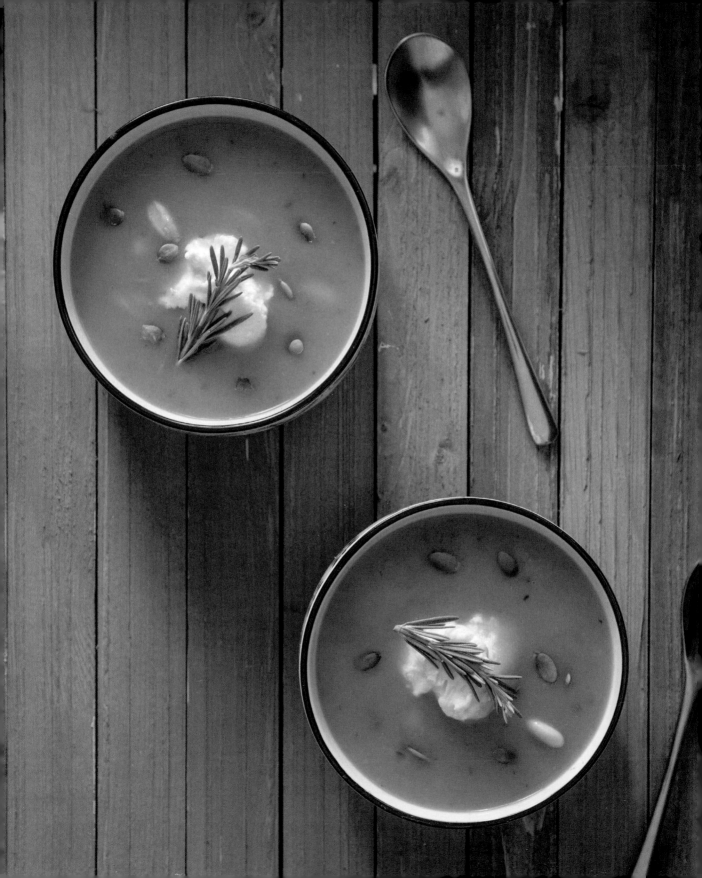

This velvety butternut and sweet potato soup is studded with creamy white beans and topped with ricotta.

Butternut and White Bean Soup

PREP TIME 10 minutes   **COOK TIME** 15 minutes   **MAKES** 4 servings   **SERVING SIZE** 1 assembled meal

NUTRITION PER SERVING Protein 21g / Carbohydrates 54g / Fiber 12g / Sugars 14g / Fat 31g / Calories 579

4 tbsp olive oil

4 garlic cloves, minced

1 small yellow onion, diced, about 5oz (150g) in total

4 sprigs fresh rosemary, chopped

1 tsp salt

3 cups water

1⅓lb (600g) diced butternut squash (about ½ small squash)

1 small sweet potato, diced, about 10½oz (300g) in total

14.5oz (425g) can cannellini beans, drained and rinsed

TO SERVE

1 cup whole-milk ricotta

8 tbsp raw pumpkin seeds

1 In a large pot, heat 2 tbsp olive oil over medium-high heat. Add the garlic, onion, rosemary, and salt. Sauté for 2 to 3 minutes, or until onion is translucent.

2 Add the butternut squash, sweet potato, and water. Bring to a boil, then reduce the heat and simmer for 10 minutes.
➥ *Return to Prep Day Action Plan while soup simmers.*

3 Using a ladle or measuring cup, carefully transfer the soup to a large blender and blend until smooth. For a thinner consistency, add more water. Work in batches if necessary.

4 To assemble the meals, divide the beans evenly among 4 containers, then ladle the puréed soup over top. Before eating, top each serving with ¼ cup ricotta and 2 tbsp pumpkin seeds.

SHOPPING LISTS

Cut the Carbs
Shopping List

Produce

- ○ 14 garlic cloves (about 2 heads of garlic)
- ○ 2 medium yellow onions
- ○ 1 red bell pepper
- ○ 4 medium zucchini squash
- ○ 1 head cauliflower, about 1¾lb (800g)
- ○ 4 cups baby arugula
- ○ 4 cups baby spinach
- ○ 2 cups fresh basil leaves, packed
- ○ 2 large lemons

Meat and Dairy

- ○ 1lb (450g) ground beef or bison
- ○ 1¼lb (600g) skinless, boneless chicken breast
- ○ 1½lb (675g) raw medium shrimp
- ○ 12 eggs
- ○ 4 tbsp butter
- ○ 16oz (450g) full-fat feta cheese
- ○ 2 tbsp shredded Parmesan
- ○ 8oz (225g) fresh mozzarella cheese

Pantry and Dry Goods

- ○ 1 cup olive oil
- ○ 1 tbsp red wine vinegar
- ○ ½ cup marinara sauce
- ○ 2 tbsp tomato paste
- ○ 2 tbsp raw almonds
- ○ 15oz (425g) can chickpeas

Spices and Seasonings

- ○ Ground cumin
- ○ Mustard powder
- ○ Smoked paprika
- ○ Parsley flakes
- ○ Red pepper flakes (optional)
- ○ Turmeric
- ○ Salt (Himalayan if possible)
- ○ Black pepper (freshly ground if possible)

TIP

Look for a low-sodium marinara sauce without added sugars.

Meal Prep Favorites
Shopping List

Produce

- 6 garlic cloves
- 1 medium yellow onion
- 1 head broccoli
- 1 bunch asparagus, about 1¼lb (600g)
- 2 cups baby spinach
- 2 medium sweet potatoes, about 10½oz (300g) total
- 2 ripe bananas
- 2 large lemons

Meat and Dairy

- 1lb (450g) ground beef
- 1½lb (675g) skinless, boneless chicken breast
- 4 skinless salmon fillets, about 4½oz (125g) each
- 2½ cups whole milk
- ½ cup full-fat Greek yogurt
- 1½ cups full-fat ricotta cheese
- 1½ cups shredded mozzarella cheese

Pantry and Dry Goods

- 6 tbsp coconut oil
- 2 tbsp hemp seeds
- 2 tbsp raw cacao powder
- 6 tbsp undenatured whey protein
- 2½ cups marinara sauce
- 1½ cups uncooked brown rice
- 1½ cups old fashioned (rolled) oats

Spices and Seasonings

- Cayenne pepper
- Ground cumin
- Dried Italian seasoning
- Dried dill
- Salt (Himalayan if possible)
- Black pepper (freshly ground if possible)

TIP
Be sure to buy plain, whole milk Greek yogurt—not vanilla.

Healthy Game Day
Shopping List

Produce

- ○ 4 garlic cloves
- ○ 3 large yellow onions
- ○ 3 red or yellow bell peppers
- ○ 2 red chili peppers, such as cayenne, about 3oz (100g) total
- ○ 2 large carrots
- ○ 3 stalks celery
- ○ 4 ripe avocados
- ○ 2 medium tomatoes
- ○ 4 tbsp chopped fresh cilantro

Meat and Dairy

- ○ 1lb (450g) ground beef
- ○ 2¼lb (1kg) skinless, boneless chicken breast
- ○ 1 tbsp crumbled blue cheese
- ○ 3oz (85g) shredded white cheddar

Pantry and Dry Goods

- ○ ½ cup olive oil, plus extra for cooking
- ○ ⅓ cup melted coconut oil
- ○ ½ cup apple cider vinegar
- ○ 1 tbsp tomato paste
- ○ 12 pitted black olives
- ○ 15oz (425g) can black beans
- ○ 8oz (220g) kidney beans (about ½ can)
- ○ 1 cup whole, raw, unsalted almonds
- ○ 1 cup whole, raw, unsalted walnuts
- ○ 1 cup pitted dates
- ○ 6 dried apricots
- ○ ¾ cup uncooked quinoa
- ○ 1 cup old fashioned (rolled) oats
- ○ ½ cup arrowroot flour
- ○ 4oz (112g) corn chips

Spices and Seasonings

- ○ Chili powder
- ○ Ground cumin
- ○ Garlic powder
- ○ Smoked paprika
- ○ Salt (Himalayan if possible)
- ○ Black pepper (freshly ground if possible)

TIP

Some oats are processed at facilities that also process wheat. Buy certified gluten-free oats if you are avoiding gluten.

Plant-Based Plates
Shopping List

Produce

- ◯ 6 garlic cloves
- ◯ 1 small yellow onion
- ◯ 1 head broccoli
- ◯ 3 red bell peppers
- ◯ 2 medium tomatoes
- ◯ 2 avocados
- ◯ 1 medium carrot
- ◯ 1 medium zucchini squash
- ◯ 4oz (100g) green beans
- ◯ 3 large mushrooms
- ◯ ¼ cup chopped fresh cilantro (optional)
- ◯ Small piece of ginger
- ◯ 12 strawberries
- ◯ 1 lime
- ◯ 2 lemons

Meat and Dairy

- ◯ 2 cups unsweetened almond milk
- ◯ 2 (12oz; 340g) packages extra-firm tofu

Pantry and Dry Goods

- ◯ ½ cup olive oil
- ◯ 2 tbsp coconut oil
- ◯ 1 tbsp red wine vinegar
- ◯ 2 tbsp tomato paste
- ◯ 2 (15oz; 425g) cans chickpeas
- ◯ 2 (15oz; 425g) cans black beans
- ◯ 1 (15oz; 425g) can lentils
- ◯ 1 (13.5oz; 398g) can full-fat coconut milk
- ◯ 6 tbsp all-natural peanut butter
- ◯ 3 tbsp chia seeds
- ◯ 1½ cups old fashioned (rolled) oats
- ◯ ¾ cup uncooked quinoa
- ◯ ½ cup uncooked basmati rice
- ◯ 4oz (112g) corn chips

Spices and Seasonings

- ◯ Chili powder
- ◯ Ground cumin
- ◯ Curry powder
- ◯ Sesame seeds
- ◯ Turmeric
- ◯ Salt (Himalayan if possible)
- ◯ Black pepper (freshly ground if possible)

TIP
Compare brands and choose an extra-firm (not silken) tofu with the most protein.

Cozy Comfort Food
Shopping List

Produce

- ○ 12 garlic cloves
- ○ 1 medium yellow onions
- ○ 6 medium zucchini squash
- ○ 3 medium sweet potatoes, about 2lb (1kg) total
- ○ 1 medium butternut squash
- ○ 8oz (250g) green beans
- ○ 2 tbsp chopped fresh rosemary
- ○ 6 bananas
- ○ 1 lemon

Meat and Dairy

- ○ 1lb (450g) ground beef
- ○ 4 skin-on, bone-in chicken thighs, about 1¼lb (600g) in total
- ○ 1¼lb (600g) skinless, boneless chicken breast
- ○ 13 eggs
- ○ ½ cup shredded cheddar cheese (optional)

Pantry and Dry Goods

- ○ ¾ cup olive oil
- ○ 6 tbsp coconut oil
- ○ 1 tbsp apple cider vinegar
- ○ 4 cups beef broth
- ○ 1 cup tomato purée
- ○ 2 tbsp tomato paste
- ○ 2 14.5oz (411g) cans diced tomatoes
- ○ 15oz (425g) can kidney beans
- ○ 4 medium pitted dates
- ○ 1 tbsp raw cacao powder
- ○ ¼ cup + 2 tbsp arrowroot flour
- ○ ½ cup coarsely ground cornmeal or polenta
- ○ 12 tbsp whey protein

Spices and Seasonings

- ○ Allspice
- ○ Cayenne pepper
- ○ Chili powder
- ○ Cinnamon
- ○ Ground cumin
- ○ Salt (Himalayan if possible)
- ○ Black pepper (freshly ground if possible)

TIP

You can use ground bison or ground turkey instead of ground beef in the chili.

Mediterranean Meals
Shopping List

Produce

- ○ 4 garlic cloves
- ○ 2 small yellow onions
- ○ 1 small red onion
- ○ 4 Roma (plum) tomatoes, about 14oz (400g) total
- ○ 2 medium tomatoes, about 14oz (400g) in total
- ○ 2 bunches asparagus
- ○ 1 medium cucumber
- ○ 1 medium zucchini squash
- ○ 1 red bell pepper
- ○ 8oz (225g) button mushrooms
- ○ 2 cups baby spinach
- ○ 2 cups chopped kale
- ○ 1 tbsp chopped fresh thyme
- ○ Handful of fresh basil leaves
- ○ 3 large lemons

Meat and Dairy

- ○ 8oz (225g) Italian sausage
- ○ 2⅔lb (1.2kg) skinless, boneless chicken breast
- ○ 4 tilapia fillets, about 4oz (125g) each
- ○ 12 eggs
- ○ ½ cup full-fat Greek yogurt
- ○ ½ cup half and half
- ○ 8oz (225g) feta cheese
- ○ 8oz (225g) full-fat mozzarella cheese

Pantry and Dry Goods

- ○ ¾ cup olive oil
- ○ 2 tbsp flaxseed oil
- ○ 2oz (60g) pitted Kalamata olives, about 20 total
- ○ ½ cup oil-packed sundried tomatoes
- ○ 8 canned artichoke hearts
- ○ ¾ cup uncooked long grain brown rice
- ○ ½ cup uncooked quinoa

Spices and Seasonings

- ○ Dried Italian seasoning
- ○ Dried oregano
- ○ Salt (Himalayan if possible)
- ○ Black pepper (freshly ground if possible)

> **TIP**
> Look for wild-caught tilapia, not farm raised. You can also use any other firm, white-fleshed fish.

Diner Delights
Shopping List

Produce

- 11 garlic cloves
- 2 medium yellow onions
- 2 sweet potatoes, about 14oz (400g) total
- 2 russet potatoes, about 1⅓lb (600g) total
- 2 heads cauliflower, about 2lb (1kg) total
- 14oz (400g) green beans
- 10oz (280g) baby spinach
- 1 tbsp chopped fresh thyme
- 1 lemon (optional)
- 3 bananas

Meat and Dairy

- 8 pork sausages, about 2½oz (75g) each
- 1½lb (700g) 90% lean ground beef
- 4 pieces cod, about 5oz (150g) each
- 2 large eggs
- 2 tbsp butter

Pantry and Dry Goods

- ¾ cup olive oil
- ½ cup + 2 tbsp coconut oil
- ¼ cup apple cider vinegar
- ¼ cup tomato paste
- 2 14.5oz (41lg) cans diced tomatoes
- 3 tbsp Dijon mustard
- 4oz (110g) whole pitted dates
- 1½ cups whole raw almonds
- ½ cup + 2 tbsp arrowroot flour
- 1½ cups undenatured whey protein
- ½ cup almond flour
- ½ cup unflavored soda water

Spices and Seasonings

- Cinnamon
- Ground cloves
- Garlic powder
- Dried Italian seasoning
- Ground nutmeg
- Onion powder
- Red pepper flakes
- Salt (Himalayan if possible)
- Black pepper (freshly ground if possible)

TIP
Buy pre-washed and pre-trimmed green beans for faster prep.

Homemade Takeout
Shopping List

Produce

- ○ 6 garlic cloves
- ○ 1 tbsp minced fresh ginger
- ○ 1lb (450g) Brussels sprouts
- ○ 2 small yellow onions
- ○ 2 bunches scallions
- ○ 5 medium carrots
- ○ 1 head broccoli
- ○ 11oz (300g) baby corn
- ○ 2 cups blueberries
- ○ ¾ cup frozen green peas

Meat and Dairy

- ○ 1¼lb (570g) pork belly
- ○ 1lb (450g) top round roast, or other inexpensive cut of beef
- ○ 1⅓lb (600g) skinless, boneless chicken breast
- ○ 2 large eggs
- ○ 1 cup whole milk
- ○ 1 cup full-fat Greek yogurt

Pantry and Dry Goods

- ○ 4 tbsp olive oil
- ○ 4 tbsp coconut oil
- ○ ¼ cup red wine vinegar
- ○ 10 tbsp coconut aminos (or liquid aminos or low-sodium soy sauce)
- ○ 2½ cups low-sodium beef stock
- ○ 15oz (425g) can black beans
- ○ 13.5oz (400ml) can coconut milk
- ○ ¾ cup chia seeds
- ○ ½ cup whey protein
- ○ 5 tbsp coconut sugar
- ○ ¼ cup + 1 tsp arrowroot flour
- ○ ¾ cup uncooked quinoa
- ○ ¾ cup uncooked brown basmati rice

Spices and Seasonings

- ○ Salt (Himalayan if possible)
- ○ Black pepper (freshly ground if possible)

TIP
If you can't find fresh baby corn, use canned.

Asian Feast
Shopping List

Produce

- ○ 8 garlic cloves
- ○ 1 small yellow onion
- ○ 1 head broccoli
- ○ 3 russet potatoes, about 1¾lb (800g) total
- ○ 1 bunch scallions
- ○ 4 red chiles, such as cayenne (optional)
- ○ Cilantro (optional, to serve)
- ○ 1in (2.5cm) piece fresh ginger
- ○ 1 lime (optional, to serve)

Meat and Dairy

- ○ 4 boneless, skinless chicken thighs
- ○ 4 skinless tilapia fillets, about 5oz (150g) each
- ○ 1lb (450g) raw, peeled, deveined shrimp
- ○ 8oz (225g) extra-firm tofu
- ○ 14 large eggs
- ○ 7 tbsp butter

Pantry and Dry Goods

- ○ ¼ cup + 2 tbsp olive oil
- ○ 5 tbsp coconut oil
- ○ 6 tbsp sesame oil
- ○ 14oz (414ml) can full-fat coconut milk
- ○ 6 tbsp low-sodium soy sauce
- ○ 2 tbsp fish sauce
- ○ 2 tbsp coconut sugar
- ○ 9oz (250g) Thai-style rice noodles
- ○ Crushed peanuts (optional, to serve)
- ○ 1¼ cups uncooked brown basmati rice

Spices and Seasonings

- ○ Ground cumin
- ○ Chili powder
- ○ Garam masala
- ○ Ground ginger
- ○ Dried Italian seasoning
- ○ Turmeric
- ○ Sesame seeds

TIP
You can use any firm-fleshed white fish in place of tilapia.

Bistro Classics
Shopping List

Produce

- ○ 6 garlic cloves
- ○ 3 medium sweet potatoes, about 1⅓lb (600g) total
- ○ 2 bunches broccolini
- ○ 2 heads cauliflower
- ○ 4 bell peppers, any color
- ○ 2 cups baby arugula
- ○ 2 cups fresh basil leaves
- ○ 2 large lemons
- ○ 1 lime
- ○ 3 cups frozen blueberries

Meat and Dairy

- ○ 4 sirloin steaks, about 5oz (150g) each
- ○ 4 pieces skinless salmon, about 4½oz (125g) each
- ○ 1⅓lb (600g) skinless, boneless chicken breast
- ○ 4 tbsp butter
- ○ 6 cups plain, full-fat Greek yogurt
- ○ 2 tbsp shredded Parmesan

Pantry and Dry Goods

- ○ ½ cup + 1 tbsp olive oil
- ○ 3 tbsp coconut oil
- ○ 1 tbsp apple cider vinegar
- ○ 1 tbsp tomato paste
- ○ 2 tbsp raw almonds
- ○ 2 tbsp arrowroot flour
- ○ ¾ cup uncooked quinoa

Spices and Seasonings

- ○ Ground cumin
- ○ Smoked paprika
- ○ Turmeric
- ○ Salt (Himalayan if possible)
- ○ Black pepper (freshly ground if possible)

Viva Variety
Shopping List

Produce

- O 7 garlic cloves
- O 1 small yellow onion
- O 2 heads bok choy
- O 1 head broccoli
- O 2 scallions
- O 4 medium zucchini squash, about 2lb (1kg) total
- O 1 bunch asparagus, about 7oz (200g)
- O 1in (2.5cm) piece fresh ginger root
- O 1 red chili pepper, such as cayenne
- O Handful of fresh basil leaves
- O 1 lemon

Meat and Dairy

- O 1⅓lb (600g) ground turkey
- O 2 skinless, boneless chicken breasts, about 1⅓lb (600g) in total
- O 13.5oz (385g) extra-firm tofu
- O 10 large eggs
- O 2 cups shredded mozzarella cheese, about 6oz (170g)
- O 8oz (225g) Camembert cheese

Pantry and Dry Goods

- O 4 tbsp olive oil
- O 7 tbsp coconut oil
- O ¼ cup apple cider vinegar
- O 3 tbsp coconut aminos (or liquid aminos)
- O 13.5oz (400ml) coconut milk
- O ¼ cup all-natural peanut butter
- O 8 oil-packed sundried tomatoes, about 2oz (50g) total
- O 2 tbsp capers
- O 3 tbsp Dijon mustard
- O ¼ cup tomato paste
- O 1½ cups uncooked long-grain brown rice
- O 1 cup polenta
- O ½ cup marinara sauce

Spices and Seasonings

- O Ground cloves
- O Garlic powder
- O Dried oregano
- O Dried rosemary
- O Red pepper flakes
- O Salt (Himalayan if possible)
- O Black pepper (freshly ground if possible)

TIP

Buy dry polenta—not the type in a tube. Substitute coarsely ground yellow cornmeal if needed.

Meatless Meals
Shopping List

Produce

- 12 garlic cloves
- 1 small yellow onion
- 1 shallot
- 2 medium eggplants
- 2 medium zucchini squash
- 1 bunch asparagus
- 8oz (225g) mushrooms
- 2 medium carrots
- 1 small butternut squash
- 1 small sweet potato
- 1 red bell pepper
- 4–5 green chili peppers, such as jalapeños
- 1in (2.5cm) piece fresh ginger root
- Handful of fresh basil leaves
- 4 sprigs fresh rosemary
- 1 bunch cilantro
- 3 ripe bananas, about 13oz (375g) total

Meat and Dairy

- 1 egg
- 2½ cups whole-milk ricotta cheese
- 2½ cups shredded full-fat mozzarella cheese

Pantry and Dry Goods

- ¼ cup olive oil
- ¼ cup melted coconut oil, plus extra for greasing
- 2 cups no-sugar-added marinara sauce
- 2 14oz (414ml) cans full-fat coconut milk
- 1 tbsp fish sauce
- 8 tbsp raw pumpkin seeds
- 2 14.5oz (425g) cans cannellini beans
- ½ tsp baking powder
- 1 tsp baking soda
- 2 tbsp coconut sugar
- ½ cup arrowroot flour
- 1 cup almond flour
- ½ cup old fashioned (rolled) oats
- 1 cup uncooked brown rice

Spices and Seasonings

- Ground cumin
- Salt (Himalayan if possible)
- Black pepper (freshly ground if possible)

Index

Entries in **bold** indicate ingredients.

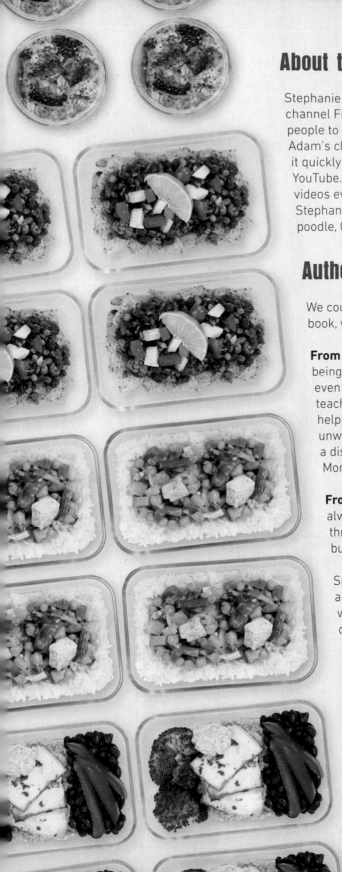

About the Authors

Stephanie Tornatore and Adam Bannon started the YouTube channel Fit Couple Cooks in 2016 with the goal of empowering people to achieve wellness goals through healthy eating. With Adam's classically trained chef skills and Stephanie's creativity, it quickly became one of the top channels for meal prep on YouTube. They continue to develop recipes and share new videos every week with hundreds of thousands of subscribers. Stephanie and Adam live in Connecticut with their miniature poodle, Giacomo Poochini.

Authors' Thanks

We could not have gotten where we are today, or written this book, without the support of our families.

From Stephanie: To Mom, Dad, and Nick—Mom, thanks for being my number-one fan and watching every single video, even when only ten other people did. Dad, thanks for teaching me how to film and edit from an early age, and for helping me develop my creativity. Thank you both for your unwavering, never-ending love...oh and um, the kitchen is a disaster right now. And Nick, you're the best present Mom and Dad ever gave me, thanks for joining us.

From Adam: Thank you to Mum, Dad, and Hayley for always supporting my big dreams, especially as I went through chef school and started my personal training business. Thanks for always telling me I could do it!

Special thank you to our extremely supportive fans from all over the world for their love and support. We wouldn't be here today without all of you sharing our content and making our recipes.

Publisher's Acknowledgments

DK/Alpha Books would like to thank the following people for their contributions.

Food stylist: Savannah Norris
Recipe testers: Josh Hohbein and Amy Thornsen
Proofreader: Laura Caddell
Indexer: Heather McNeill

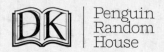

Publisher Mike Sanders
Associate publisher Billy Fields
Editor Ann Barton
Book designer and art director William Thomas
Photographer Kelley Jordan
Prepress technician Brian Massey

First American Edition, 2017
Published in the United States by DK Publishing
6081 E. 82nd Street, Indianapolis, Indiana 46250

Copyright © 2017 Dorling Kindersley Limited
A Penguin Random House Company
17 18 19 20   10 9 8 7 6 5 4 3 2 1
01–306713–Dec/2017

Published in the United States by Dorling Kindersley Limited.

ISBN: 978-1-4654-6486-6

Library of Congress Catalog Number: 2017933255

Note: This publication contains the opinions and ideas of its author(s). It is
intended to provide helpful and informative material on the subject matter
covered. It is sold with the understanding that the author(s) and publisher
are not engaged in rendering professional services in the book. If the
reader requires personal assistance or advice, a competent professional
should be consulted. The author(s) and publisher specifically disclaim any
responsibility for any liability, loss, or risk, personal or otherwise, which is
incurred as a consequence, directly or indirectly, of the use and application
of any of the contents of this book.

Trademarks: All terms mentioned in this book that are known to be or are
suspected of being trademarks or service marks have been appropriately
capitalized. Alpha Books, DK, and Penguin Random House LLC cannot
attest to the accuracy of this information. Use of a term in this book should
not be regarded as affecting the validity of any trademark or service mark.

DK books are available at special discounts when purchased in bulk for
sales promotions, premiums, fund-raising, or educational use. For details,
contact: DK Publishing Special Markets, 345 Hudson Street, New York, New
York 10014 or SpecialSales@dk.com.

Printed and bound in China

A WORLD OF IDEAS:
SEE ALL THERE IS TO KNOW
www.dk.com

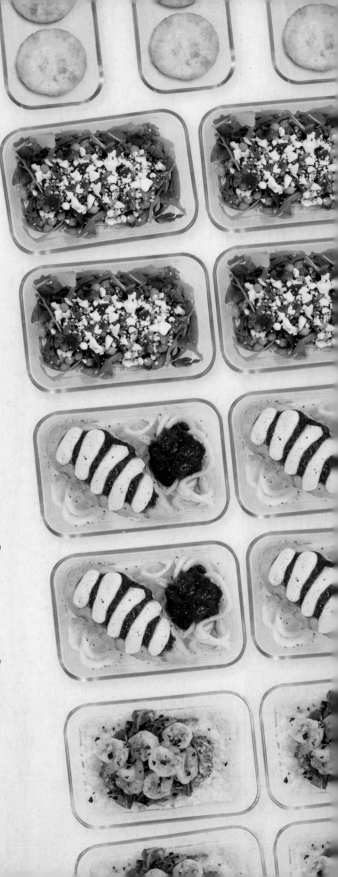